A Public Health Action Plan to Prevent Heart Disease and Stroke

CONTENTS

EXECUTIVE SUMMARY

Purpose of the plan: To chart a course for the Centers for Disease Control and Prevention (CDC) and collaborating public health agencies, with all interested partners and the public at large, to help in promoting achievement of national goals for preventing heart disease and stroke over the next two decades—through 2020 and beyond.

Heart disease and stroke are among the nation's leading causes of death and major causes of disability, projected to cost more than $351 billion in 2003. In the next two decades, these conditions can be expected to increase sharply as this country's "baby boom" generation ages. The current disease burden, recent trends, and growing disparities among certain populations reinforce this projection.

Yet these conditions are largely preventable. As expressed in the *Steps to a HealthierUS* initiative from Secretary of Health and Human Services Tommy G. Thompson, the long-term solution for our nation's health care crisis requires embracing prevention as the first step. To reverse the epidemic of heart disease and stroke through increasingly effective prevention, action is needed now.

A Public Health Action Plan to Prevent Heart Disease and Stroke addresses this urgent need for action. Key partners, public health experts, and heart disease and stroke prevention specialists came together to develop targeted recommendations and specific action steps toward achievement of this goal, through a process convened by CDC and its parent agency, the U.S. Department of Health and Human Services (HHS).

CDC and public health partners will provide national leadership to assure meaningful progress in implementing the plan. This includes bringing the public health community together with new and existing partners representing every interested segment of society. An important aspect of this process is continuing coordination between CDC and the National Institutes of Health (NIH), HHS, which is the co-lead agency with CDC for the heart disease and stroke focus area of *Healthy People 2010*.

Today, support for public health programs to prevent heart disease and stroke remains low, constituting less than 3% of the aggregate budget of our state public health agencies. Despite substantial public health gains in recent years, the failure to halt and reverse the epidemic has been extremely costly. Numbers of victims and health care expenses will only escalate unless the epidemic is reversed.

Fortunately, a new promise of success exists today. We have knowledge from decades of research and experience, especially because of the contributions of NIH and the American Heart Association. We also have a growing commitment to prevention, exemplified by the Secretary's *Steps to a HealthierUS* initiative. And we have the potential collaboration of many major national partners.

The *Action Plan* represents a comprehensive public health strategy to assist in addressing the *Healthy People 2010* goal of improving cardiovascular health through the prevention, detection, and treatment of risk factors; early identification and treatment of heart attacks and strokes; and prevention of recurrent cardiovascular events. This strategy depends on a balanced investment in all available intervention approaches, from policy and environmental changes designed to prevent risk factors to assurance of quality care for the victims of heart disease and stroke, and it includes education to support individual efforts to prevent or control risk factors.

To successfully implement the plan, two fundamental requirements must be met. First, we must communicate to the public at large and to policy makers the urgent need and unprecedented opportunity to prevent heart disease and stroke. Second, we must transform the nation's public health infrastructure to provide leadership and to develop and maintain effective partnerships and collaborations to support the needed actions.

The five essential components of this plan are taking action, strengthening capacity, evaluating impact, advancing policy, and engaging in regional and global partnerships. In these five areas, 22 recommendations and supporting action steps are proposed for implementation over the course of this long-term plan. In summary form, these recommendations are as follows:

• Develop new policies in accordance with advances in science and implement new intervention programs in a timely manner in multiple settings, for all age groups, for whole populations, and especially for high-risk groups, on a scale sufficient to have measurable impacts.

• Strengthen public health agencies and create training opportunities, model standards, and resources for continuous technical support for these agencies and their partners.

• Enhance data sources and systems to monitor key indicators relevant to heart disease and stroke prevention and to systematically evaluate policy and program interventions.

• Foster research on policies and public health programs aimed at preventing atherosclerosis and high blood pressure, especially at the community level. Continue to evaluate the public health role of genetic and other biomarkers of risk. Develop innovative ways to evaluate public health interventions, particularly those related to policy and environmental change and population-wide health promotion.

• Work with regional and global partners to reap the full benefit of sharing knowledge and experience in heart disease and stroke prevention with these partners.

The next step is to develop a detailed implementation plan—first setting priorities, then assessing the potential alignment of proposed action steps with the interests of individual partners, adopting short- and long-term time lines, and formulating feasible approaches for evaluation. CDC is committed to providing leadership and support to convene these ongoing efforts, inviting all interested partners to collaborate in action areas congruent with their own interests.

OVERVIEW

Heart disease and stroke are epidemic in the United States and elsewhere.[1,2] In the next two decades, these largely preventable conditions are projected to increase sharply in numbers as this country's "baby boom" generation ages.[3,4] The message is urgent—action is needed now to reverse the epidemic of heart disease and stroke.

A Comprehensive Public Health Strategy

Effective action will require a comprehensive public health strategy and a sustained commitment to its implementation. *A Public Health Action Plan to Prevent Heart Disease and Stroke* addresses these requirements. CDC invited participants to develop the plan, in keeping with its responsibility for undertaking activities to help move the nation toward achievement of the goal for heart disease and stroke prevention under *Healthy People 2010*.[5]

This followed designation of CDC as co-lead agency for this focus area, joining the National Institutes of Health (NIH), which had sole responsibility for this area previously. NIH, with CDC and other partners, participated in the Working Group that guided the planning process. In addition, public health experts and heart disease and stroke prevention specialists in the United States and abroad were asked to participate in the Working Group, one of five Expert Panels, or a National Forum.

For the Expert Panels, each of which was chaired by an extramural public health expert, 45 national and international experts contributed to formulation of the recommendations and proposed action steps. For the Working Group, which also was chaired by an extramural public health expert, 20 national and international experts served. For the National Forum, which was presided over by the chair of the Working Group, 81 individuals representing 66 national and international organizations and agencies other than CDC participated. With technical support from CDC, these groups developed the substance of the plan. These activities occurred from December 2001 through September 2002.

The resulting plan belongs to all who wish to use it. For successful implementation, public health agencies and the overall public health community must join with new and existing partners representing every interested segment of society. CDC and other public health agencies will provide leadership for working with partners to assure that meaningful progress is made. Participation is welcomed from all who wish to contribute. Continuing collaboration with NIH as co-lead agency will be important.

The Challenge

Despite the major progress in reducing death rates from heart disease and stroke, their total impact has increased in the past 50 years according to many health status indicators.[1,6] In the United States, growing

Every 29 seconds, someone will suffer a coronary event in the United States. Every 60 seconds, someone will die from such an event.

Every 45 seconds, someone will suffer a new or recurrent stroke. Every 3.1 minutes, someone will die from a stroke.

Many people believe that cardiovascular disease only affects men and older people. But heart disease and stroke are among the leading causes of death for U.S. women and men in all racial and ethnic groups, and sudden cardiac deaths have increased dramatically among people younger than age 35.

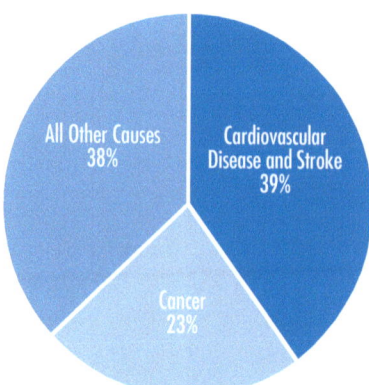

All Other Causes 38%

Cardiovascular Disease and Stroke 39%

Cancer 23%

Causes of Death for all Americans in the United States, 2000

In 2002, CDC funded cardiovascular disease prevention programs in 29 states and the District of Columbia. The Heart Disease and Stroke Prevention Program is designed to reduce disparities in treatment, risk factors, and disease; delay the onset of disease; postpone death; and reduce disabling conditions. The goal is a national program with sufficient funding for every state.

**CDC Funding
for State Programs
Fiscal Year 2002**

☐ No CDC Funding
▨ Funding for Capacity Building
◼ Funding for Basic Implementation

☐ DE
  MD
  NH
  NJ
  RI
  VT

▨ CT
  DC
  MA

numbers of people are dying from these conditions or surviving with disability, dependency, and high risk for recurrence. During the 1990s, although the overall death rate for these conditions declined 17.0%, the actual number of deaths increased 2.5%. This reflects, in part, growth in the population over age 65, which has the highest rates and therefore contributes most to the mounting numbers of deaths each year.[7]

As a result, heart disease remained the nation's leading cause of death in 2000 for women and men and for nearly every racial and ethnic group. Stroke is the third leading cause of death, and both conditions are major causes of disability for people 65 and older, as well as for many younger adults. Thus, the importance of these conditions is not restricted to the older population, though the number of victims at older ages are especially great. Risk factors such as diabetes have increased sharply, even for younger people.[8] Growing health disparities place certain populations, especially racial or ethnic minorities and people of low income or education, at excess risk relative to groups with the most favorable rates of heart disease and stroke.[9–12] Aging of the baby boom generation portends a sharp rise by 2020 in the number of people who die from heart disease and stroke or survive with dependency.[3,4]

Clearly, heart disease and stroke contribute substantially to the nation's health care crisis, as addressed by Secretary of Health and Human Services Tommy G. Thompson in his initiative, *Steps to a HealthierUS*. This initiative places an important new emphasis on prevention of chronic diseases and conditions.

The epidemic of heart disease and stroke can be expected to continue, with an increasing burden and widening disparities, unless unprecedented public health efforts are mounted to arrest and reverse it. This challenge will test the ability of public health institutions at all levels to fulfill their obligation to protect society against this rising epidemic. Three factors affect the current challenge.

- **Support for public health programs to prevent heart disease and stroke is low.** State public health agencies expend less than 3% of their budgets on chronic disease programs, including heart disease and stroke prevention.[7]
- **The costs of failure are very high.** The economic costs of heart disease and stroke rise each year. These costs include the numbers of people requiring treatment for risk factors or early signs of disease; emergency treatment for first or recurrent episodes of heart attack, heart failure, or stroke; and efforts to reduce disability and prevent recurrent episodes. In 2003, health care costs alone are projected to be $209.3 billion. Although personal and societal costs are incalculable, they include another $142.5 billion in lost productivity.[1] These costs will escalate further if this epidemic is not halted and reversed. As noted by Secretary Thompson, chronic diseases and conditions, including heart disease, consume more than 75% of our nation's health care dollars, yet they are largely preventable.
- **An unprecedented opportunity to prevent heart disease and stroke exists today in the United States.** We know what causes

these conditions and how to prevent them, largely because of the decades of research supported by NIH, the American Heart Association, and others.[6] *Healthy People 2010* has outlined clear goals, and the Healthy People 2010 Heart and Stroke Partnership* was established to help in achieving them.[5] Also, health professionals have become more aware of the need for immediate action as they increasingly recognize the continuing cardiovascular epidemic, recent unfavorable trends, and forecasts of a mounting disease burden.[8]

The Public Health Response

Substantial public health achievements have been made in preventing heart disease and stroke, but they are insufficient to arrest or reverse the epidemic. Public health serves society by guaranteeing conditions of life in which people can be healthy and by addressing three core functions—assessment, policy development, and assurance.[13] Achievements in these areas as they relate to heart disease and stroke[6] include the following:

- **Assessment.** For several decades, public health agencies and researchers have collected data on the epidemic and conducted research on how to control it. Although important gaps persist, the accumulated knowledge provides a solid evidence base for public health decision making.
- **Policy development.** A wealth of policies has been developed on the basis of this knowledge. Some policies have been implemented effectively but await broader, more intensive application to achieve their full impact. Others have yet to be acted upon. Evaluating these policies requires implementation on a sufficient scale and adequate resources for evaluation.
- **Assurance.** Assurance, measured by how much society is protected from epidemic heart disease and stroke, remains to be achieved despite recent progress. Public health agencies can put current knowledge to work through a targeted plan of action. Unfortunately, most public health agencies are not yet well-equipped for this task.[13]

The U.S. Department of Health and Human Services (HHS) and its component agencies, including NIH and especially its National Heart, Lung, and Blood Institute and National Institute of Neurological Disorders and Stroke, represent a long history of research and program development in the area of heart disease and stroke for both health professionals and the public. It is beyond the scope of this document to inventory the contributions of even one agency, much less those of HHS as a whole, but it is important to recognize that today's knowledge base about prevention of heart disease and stroke is, to a large degree, a reflection of this work. Other organizations, especially the American Heart Association, also have supported research that has led to the kinds of policy developments—often in partnership with others, such as the American College of Cardiology—that underlie the present opportunity

The *Steps to a HealthierUS* initiative envisions a healthy, strong United States where diseases are prevented when possible, controlled when necessary, and treated when appropriate. This initiative is a bold shift in our approach to the health of our citizens, moving us from a disease care system to a health care system. We can no longer sustain the skyrocketing health care costs created by an over reliance on treatment, nor should Americans continue to suffer from preventable diseases.

---

* Current partners include the American Heart Association/American Stroke Association, CDC, Centers for Medicare & Medicaid Services, Indian Health Service, NIH, and Office of Public Health and Science, U.S. Department of Health and Human Services.

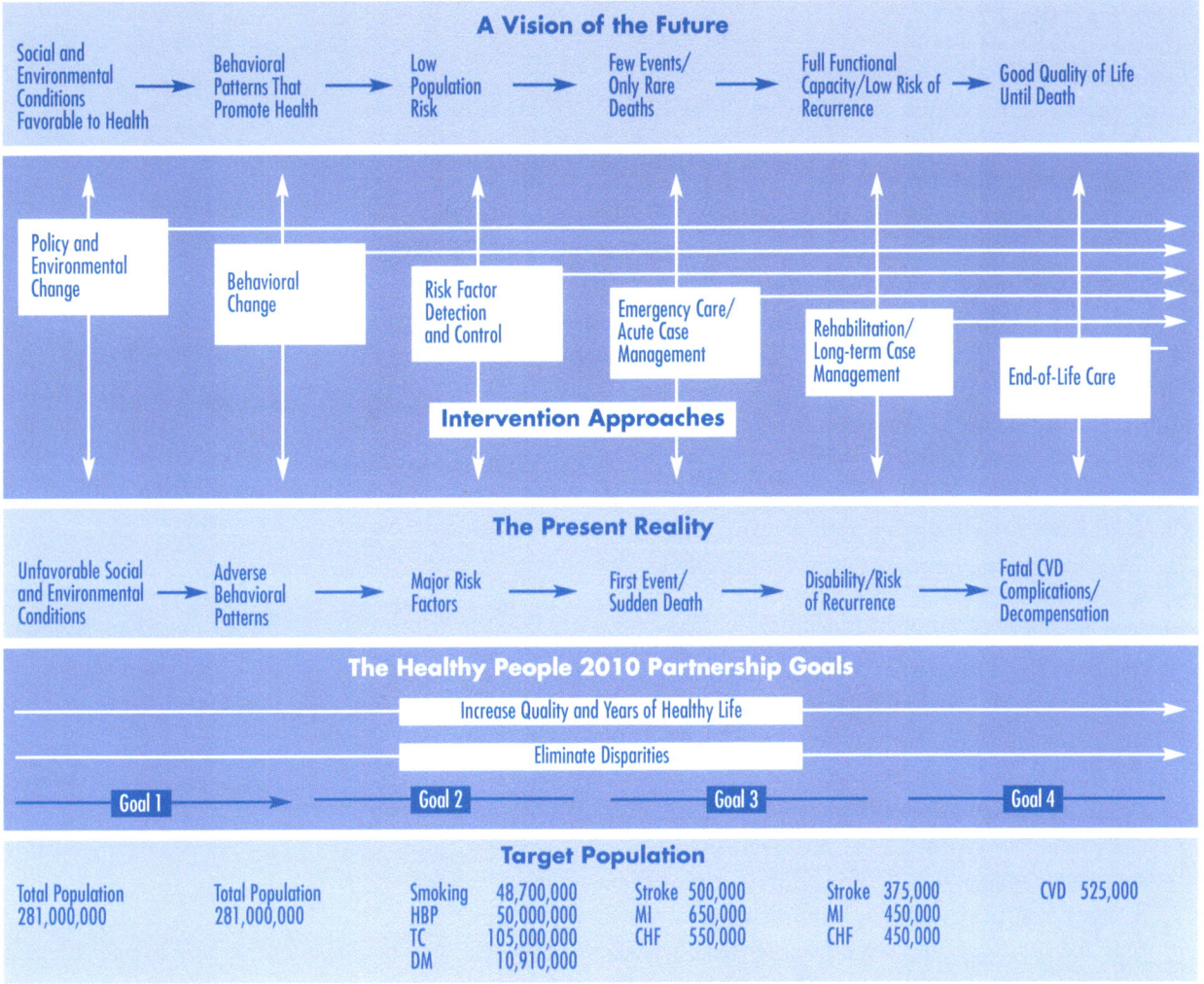

A Vision of the Future

Social and Environmental Conditions Favorable to Health → Behavioral Patterns That Promote Health → Low Population Risk → Few Events/ Only Rare Deaths → Full Functional Capacity/Low Risk of Recurrence → Good Quality of Life Until Death

Policy and Environmental Change

Behavioral Change

Risk Factor Detection and Control

Emergency Care/ Acute Case Management

Rehabilitation/ Long-term Case Management

End-of-Life Care

Intervention Approaches

The Present Reality

Unfavorable Social and Environmental Conditions → Adverse Behavioral Patterns → Major Risk Factors → First Event/ Sudden Death → Disability/Risk of Recurrence → Fatal CVD Complications/ Decompensation

The Healthy People 2010 Partnership Goals

Increase Quality and Years of Healthy Life

Eliminate Disparities

Goal 1   Goal 2   Goal 3   Goal 4

Target Population

Total Population 281,000,000	Total Population 281,000,000	Smoking 48,700,000 HBP 50,000,000 TC 105,000,000 DM 10,910,000	Stroke 500,000 MI 650,000 CHF 550,000	Stroke 375,000 MI 450,000 CHF 450,000	CVD 525,000

Note: Healthy People 2010 goals are explained in the text. HBP = high blood pressure, TC = total cholesterol, DM = diabetes mellitus, MI = myocardial infarction, CHF = congestive heart failure, CVD = cardiovascular disease.

Figure 1. Action Framework for a Comprehensive Public Health Strategy to Prevent Heart Disease and Stroke (see the inside back cover for a color version of this figure)

for heart disease and stroke prevention. CDC has contributed in this area for many years through its laboratory standardization, surveillance, and vital statistics activities, as well as through more recent public health program implementation.

In the context of this HHS tradition, Secretary Thompson's *Steps to a HealthierUS* initiative is a significant new development. It calls for marshalling all available resources within HHS and for action by other federal agencies, such as transportation, agriculture, and education, and private-sector interests, such as the food industry and many others. All are urged to take steps to improve the nation's health. Further, this initiative calls on policy makers to embrace prevention as the first step toward solving our nation's health care crisis. Clearly, it is understood that business as usual will not be sufficient to meet today's challenges in addressing chronic diseases and conditions, including heart disease and stroke.

The *Action Plan*

The *Action Plan* embraces the two overarching goals of *Healthy People 2010*, which are to increase quality and years of healthy life and to eliminate health disparities.[5] It also addresses four goals specific to heart disease and stroke, as distinguished by the Healthy People 2010 Heart and Stroke Partnership according to the different intervention approaches that apply. These goals (which are based on the one *Healthy People 2010* goal) are prevention of risk factors, detection and treatment of risk factors, early identification and treatment of heart attacks and strokes, and prevention of recurrent cardiovascular events. An action framework that outlines the comprehensive public health strategy of the *Action Plan* (see Figure 1) highlights these goals. The main features of the action framework can be described briefly as follows (see full report for further discussion):

- **The Present Reality**, which summarizes current knowledge of the progressive development of heart disease and stroke.
- **A Vision of the Future**, which summarizes the favorable circumstances that must be achieved if the epidemic of heart disease and stroke is to be arrested and reversed.
- **Intervention Approaches**, which include the six broad approaches that, when fully and effectively implemented, can help bring about the transition to the vision of the future.
- **Healthy People 2010 Partnership Goals** for reducing heart disease and stroke and how the six intervention approaches can address successive stages of disease and help attain these goals.
- **Target Population**, which indicates how many people could be reached by each successive intervention approach.

This public health strategy is based on the concept of pursuing the *Healthy People 2010* goal for preventing heart disease and stroke by applying the full array of intervention approaches. For this *Action Plan*, participants proposed specific recommendations after identifying public health areas critical to preventing heart disease and stroke. Five such areas were established as essential components of the plan (see Figure 2, next page). For each component, CDC convened an Expert Panel to consider the relevant issues and recommend action steps through which to address them. Detailed implementation plans will be developed in each area subsequently, guided by the overall plan.

The five components and their respective panels are summarized as follows:

- **Taking action**. Translating current knowledge into effective public health action (Expert Panel A).
- **Strengthening capacity.** Transforming public health agencies with new competencies and resources and expanding partnerships to mount and sustain such action (Expert Panel B).
- **Evaluating impact.** Systematically monitoring and evaluating the health impact of interventions to identify and rapidly disseminate those most effective (Expert Panel C).

"We have the scientific knowledge to create a world in which most cardiovascular disease could be eliminated."

From *The 2000 Victoria Declaration on Women, Heart Diseases and Stroke*

The Utah Cardiovascular Health Program partnered with 140 organizations representing government, private businesses, health care organizations, and nonprofit agencies to form the Alliance for Cardiovascular Health. This group has developed a 3-year plan to identify key strategies for improving cardiovascular health, including policy and environmental change.

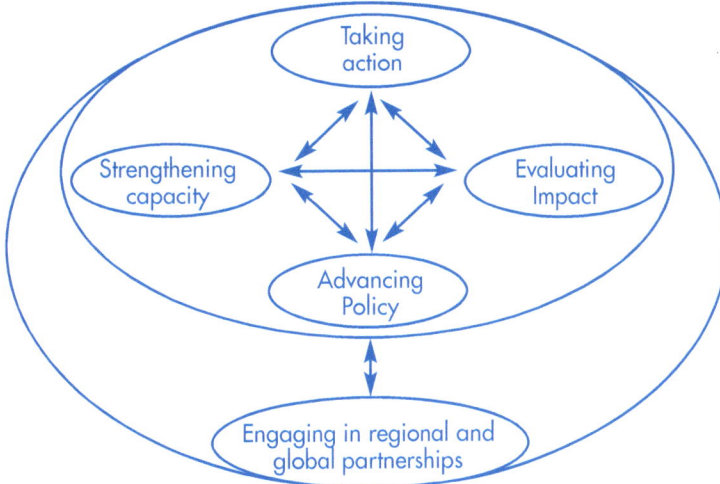

Figure 2. An Integrated Action Plan to Prevent Heart Disease and Stroke

- **Advancing policy.** Defining the most critical policy issues and pursuing the needed prevention research to resolve them and expedite policy development (Expert Panel D).
- **Engaging in regional and global partnerships.** Multiplying resources and capitalizing on shared experience with others throughout the global community who are addressing similar challenges (Expert Panel E).

The Expert Panels proposed specific recommendations and action steps for implementing the plan over the next two decades and beyond. For this Overview, the full list of recommendations was synthesized into two fundamental requirements and 10 summary recommendations.

Fundamental Requirements

- **We must communicate to the public at large and to policy makers the urgent need and unprecedented opportunity to prevent heart disease and stroke in order to establish wide-spread awareness and concern about these conditions, as well as confidence in the ability to prevent and control them.**

An effective, comprehensive public health strategy to prevent heart disease and stroke depends on widespread understanding of three basic messages. Heart disease and stroke threaten the health and well-being of all Americans, especially during the middle and older adult years. Prevention is possible by reversing community-acquired behaviors, risks, and health disparities. Failure to intensify preventive efforts now will sharply escalate the future burden and cost of these conditions. To effectively implement this plan, we must communicate these and other clear messages through appropriate channels, with support from appropriate partners. A communications infrastructure is needed that includes public health agencies at all levels, tribal and other governmental agencies, the private sector (e.g., voluntary and faith-based associations, professional and business groups, media, foundations), and broad community participation.

African Americans are more adversely affected by heart disease and stroke than any other racial group in the United States. To combat this disparity, the Association of Black Cardiologists is conducting a public education campaign called *Children Should Know Their Grandparents: A Guide to a Healthy Heart*. This program encourages healthy lifestyle choices to prevent heart disease and stroke and stresses the importance of sharing family medical histories.

• **We must transform the nation's public health infrastructure to provide leadership and to develop and maintain effective partnerships and collaborations for the action needed.**

Such changes, which will be elaborated in a detailed implementation plan, will enable public health leaders to bring together the array of partners needed to prevent heart disease and stroke. These changes will also lead public health agencies to recognize and aggressively emphasize the policy and environmental changes and population-wide information and education needed for health behavior change.

Summary Recommendations

1. **Develop policies for preventing heart disease and stroke at national, state, and local levels to assure effective public health action, including new knowledge on the efficacy and safety of therapies to reduce risk factors. Implement intervention programs in a timely manner and on a sufficient scale to permit rigorous evaluation and the rapid replication and dissemination of those most effective.**

Active intervention is needed continually to develop and support policies (both in and beyond the health sector) that are favorable to health, change those that are unfavorable, and foster policy innovations when gaps are identified. Policies that adversely affect health should be identified because they can be major barriers to the social, environmental, and behavioral changes needed to improve population-wide health.

2. **Promote cardiovascular health and prevent heart disease and stroke through interventions in multiple settings, for all age groups, and for the whole population, especially high-risk groups.**

This recommendation defines the scope of a comprehensive public health strategy to prevent heart disease and stroke. Such a strategy must 1) emphasize promotion of desirable social and environmental conditions and favorable population-wide and individual behavioral patterns to prevent major risk factors and 2) assure full accessibility and timely use of quality health services among people with risk factors or disease.

3. **Strengthen public health agencies to assure that they develop and maintain sufficient capacities and competencies, including their laboratories.**

Public health agencies at state and local levels should establish specific programs designed to promote cardiovascular health and prevent heart disease and stroke. Skills are required in the new priority areas of policy and environmental change, population-wide health promotion through behavioral change, and risk factor prevention. Public

"At no time in the history of this nation has the mission of promoting and protecting the public's health resonated more clearly with the public and the government than now. To improve health in our communities, we need high-quality and well-educated public health professionals."

From *Who Will Keep the Public Healthy? Educating Public Health Professionals for the 21st Century*, Institute of Medicine, 2002

"To reach minority populations, the American Heart Association created Search Your Heart. This faith-based program is established primarily in the inner cities for the medically underserved, high-risk segment of our population. Important cardiovascular health messages are delivered through the 5,000 places of worship enrolled in this program nationwide."

Robert O. Bonow, MD, President, American Heart Association

The Oklahoma Cardiovascular Health Program has developed rules to help emergency and hospital workers better serve stroke patients, based on American Heart Association and National Stroke Association guidelines.

The state-based Behavioral Risk Factor Surveillance System (BRFSS) is the largest telephone survey tool in the world. Data have been collected on the public's knowledge of the signs and symptoms of heart attack and stroke, their access to and participation in health care, and other issues related to quality of life. BRFSS data help health care professionals and policy makers effectively address the needs of specific populations and geographic areas.

health agencies must also be able to manage and use health data systems to effectively monitor and evaluate interventions and prevention programs. Laboratory capacity and standardization must be maintained to address new and continuing demands and opportunities.

4. **Create opportunities for training, offer model standards for preventing chronic diseases, and make consultation and technical support continuously available to public health agencies, including their laboratories.**

This plan demands new skills and competencies that can only be met through new training opportunities (see full document for details). Public health agencies can fulfill their responsibilities and function effectively in the new era of diverse partnerships by taking advantage of these opportunities.

5. **Define criteria and standards for population-wide health data sources. Expand these sources as needed to assure adequate long-term monitoring of population measures related to heart disease and stroke.**

Such measures include mortality, incidence, and prevalence rates; selected biomarkers of CVD risk; risk factors and behaviors; economic conditions; community and environmental characteristics; sociodemographic factors (e.g., age, race/ethnicity, sex, place of residence); and leading health indicators. Appropriate criteria and standards can be defined through a national meeting of key stakeholders. In addition, they must conform to the National Health Information Infrastructure (www.health.gov/ncvhs-nhii) and the Standards for Privacy of Individually Identifiable Health Information, also called the Privacy Rule (www.hhs.gov/ocr/hipaa).

6. **Upgrade and expand health data sources to allow systematic monitoring and evaluation of policy and program interventions.**

To learn what works best, all programs funded by public health agencies should allocate resources for evaluation upfront, and staff must be trained to develop and apply evaluation methods. The resulting data must be communicated effectively to other agencies and to policy makers.

7. **Emphasize the critical roles of atherosclerosis and high blood pressure, which are the dominant conditions underlying heart disease and stroke, within a broad prevention research agenda.**

Prevention research on policy, environmental, and sociocultural determinants of risk factors, as well as potentially useful genetic and other biomarkers of risk, is critical, as is rapid translation of this information into health care practice. Policy makers must understand the value of such research. Such research should focus especially on children and adolescents because atherosclerosis and high blood pressure can begin early in life. The prevention research agenda should be developed and updated collaboratively among interested parties, taking current and planned research programs into account.

8. **Develop innovative ways to monitor and evaluate policies and programs, especially for policy and environmental change and population-wide health promotion.**

   Public health agencies and their partners should conduct and promote research to improve surveillance methods in multiple areas, settings, and populations. Marketing research can be used to evaluate public knowledge and awareness of key health messages and to update these messages over time. Methodological research can help assess the impact of new technologies and regulations on surveillance systems.

9. **Reap the full benefit of shared knowledge and experience from regional and global partners through information exchange in the area of heart disease and stroke prevention.**

   Such communication will promote productive interactions among public health agencies in the United States and their counterparts elsewhere in the world addressing similar challenges. As a result, this nation will benefit from the investment of others by gaining valuable knowledge and experience in public health approaches to heart disease and stroke prevention.

10. **Work with regional and global partners to develop prevention policies, formulate strategies for use of global media for health communications, and assess the impact of globalization on cardiovascular health.**

    With these partners, the U.S. public health community can explore new ways to enhance the skills and resources of global health agencies, apply new methods for monitoring and evaluating interventions, and further research by fostering replication of studies in diverse settings.

Implementation

Immediate action is needed to prevent heart disease and stroke. To initiate and sustain this action, commitment is needed from national, state, and local public health agencies; tribal organizations; and others within and beyond the health sector. Implementation of the *Action Plan* should complement other activities in pursuit of the *Healthy People 2010* goal for preventing heart disease and stroke and be appropriately coordinated with the existing Healthy People 2010 Heart and Stroke Partnership. The complete *Action Plan* can be reviewed at www.cdc.gov/cvh.

References

1. American Heart Association. *Heart and Stroke Statistics—2003 Update*. Dallas, TX: American Heart Association; 2003.

2. Murray CJL, Lopez A. Alternative Projections of Mortality and Disability by Cause 1990–2020: Global Burden of Disease Study. *Lancet* 1997;349:1498–1504.

3. Foot DK, Lewis RP, Pearson TA, Beller GA. Demographics and Cardiology, 1950–2050. *Journal of the American College of Cardiology* 2000;35(No. 5, Suppl B):66B–80B.

4. Howard G, Howard VJ. Stroke Incidence, Mortality, and Prevalence. In: Gorelick PB, Alter M, editors. *The Prevention of Stroke*. New York, NY: The Parthenon Publishing Group; 2002:1–10.

5. US Department of Health and Human Services. *Healthy People 2010: Understanding and Improving Health and Objectives for Improving Health*. 2nd ed. Vol 1. Washington, DC: US Government Printing Office; November 2000.

6. Labarthe DR. *Epidemiology and Prevention of Cardiovascular Diseases: A Global Challenge*. Gaithersburg, MD: Aspen Publishers; 1998.

7. Centers for Disease Control and Prevention. *Unrealized Prevention Opportunities: Reducing the Health and Economic Burden of Chronic Disease*. Atlanta, GA: US Department of Health and Human Services, Centers for Disease Control and Prevention; 2000.

8. Cooper R, Cutler J, Desvigne-Nickens P, et al. Trends and Disparities in Coronary Heart Disease, Stroke, and Other Cardiovascular Diseases in the United States. Findings of the National Conference on Cardiovascular Disease Prevention. *Circulation* 2000;102:3137–47.

9. Centers for Disease Control and Prevention. *Health, United States, 2002. With Chartbook on Trends in the Health of Americans*. Hyattsville, MD: US Department of Health and Human Services, Centers for Disease Control and Prevention; 2002. DHHS publication no. 1232.

10. Casper ML, Barnett E, Halverson JA, et al. *Women and Heart Disease: An Atlas of Racial and Ethnic Disparities in Mortality. Second Edition*. Morgantown, WV: Office for Social Environment and Health Research; 2000.

11. Barnett E, Casper ML, Halverson JA, et al. *Men and Heart Disease: An Atlas of Racial and Ethnic Disparities in Mortality. First Edition*. Morgantown, WV: Office for Social Environment and Health Research; 2001.

12. Casper ML, Barnett E, Williams GI Jr, et al. *Atlas of Stroke Mortality: Racial, Ethnic, and Geographic Disparities in the United States*. Atlanta, GA: US Department of Health and Human Services, Centers for Disease Control and Prevention; January 2003.

13. Committee for the Study of the Future of Public Health, Division of Health Care Services, Institute of Medicine. *The Future of Public Health*. Washington, DC: National Academy Press; 1988.

SECTION 1.
HEART DISEASE AND STROKE PREVENTION: TIME FOR ACTION

Summary

The continuing epidemic of cardiovascular diseases (CVD) in the United States and globally calls for renewed and intensified public health action to prevent heart disease and stroke. Public health agencies at national, state, and local levels (including CDC in partnership with NIH) bear a special responsibility to meet this call, along with tribal organizations and all other interested partners. The widespread occurrence and silent progression of atherosclerosis and high blood pressure (the dominant conditions underlying heart disease and stroke) has created a CVD burden that is massive in terms of its attendant death, disability, and social and economic costs. This burden is projected to increase sharply by 2020 because of the changing age structure of the U.S. population and other factors, including the rising prevalence of obesity and diabetes. Several popular myths and misconceptions have obscured this reality, and these must be dispelled through effective communication with the public at large and with policy makers.

More than a half-century of research and experience has provided a strong scientific basis for preventing heart disease and stroke. Policy statements and guidelines for prevention have been available for more than four decades and have increased in breadth, depth, and number to guide both public health action and clinical practice. National public health goals have been updated to 2010 and include a specific call to prevent heart disease and stroke. Achieving this goal would greatly accelerate progress toward achieving the nation's two overarching health goals—increasing quality and years of healthy life and eliminating health disparities. CVD is a major contributor to early death (measured as years of life lost) and to differences in life expectancy among racial and ethnic groups.

An unprecedented opportunity exists today to develop and implement an effective public health strategy to prevent heart disease and stroke. Three major factors have contributed to this opportunity:

- More cumulative knowledge and experience in CVD prevention exists today than ever before.
- Major national partnerships have been established to support heart disease and stroke prevention.
- Health professionals increasingly recognize the continuing CVD epidemic, unfavorable recent trends, and forecasts of a mounting burden of heart disease and stroke, nationally and worldwide. This recognition has increased their awareness of the need for immediate action.

Despite this opportunity, the public health investment in preventing heart disease and stroke remains far below what is needed for fully effective intervention. Serious shortcomings also exist in the delivery of established treatments for these conditions in clinical practice. These facts demonstrate that the vast body of current knowledge and experience in CVD prevention has yet to be adequately applied to realize the full potential benefit to the public's health. The most critical need today is for public health action that is guided by the knowledge and experience already at hand.

Introduction: Planning for the Prevention of Heart Disease and Stroke

Heart disease and stroke together exact a greater toll on America's health than any other condition.[1] Early death, disability, personal and family disruption, loss of income (more than $142 billion for 2003), and medical care expenditures (more than $209 billion) are some indicators of this toll. Young and old, women and men, rich and poor, and all racial and ethnic groups share this burden. Moreover, we can expect even greater numbers of heart attacks and strokes, increasing dependency (especially among the expanding population of older Americans), and mounting costs of care for victims and their families unless we as a nation renew and greatly intensify our public health effort to prevent these conditions.

Heart attacks and strokes can be prevented or delayed if the knowledge we already have is put into action now. In fact, a broad coalition of national organizations and federal health agencies have already adopted a comprehensive goal for preventing heart disease and stroke as part of the *Healthy People 2010* national health goals.[2] But having goals is only a beginning. Attaining these goals requires a plan with specific recommendations and action steps for implementing them. Today, we can build such an action plan on a solid knowledge base resulting from decades of research on the causes and prevention of heart disease and stroke, especially because of the support of NIH and the American Heart Association.

For CDC, developing an action plan for cardiovascular health (CVH) is critical for two compelling reasons. First, CDC and NIH have been assigned responsibility as co-lead agencies to head the nation's effort to attain the *Healthy People 2010* goal for preventing heart disease and stroke.[2] Second, Congress charged CDC in 1998 to develop and implement state-based cardiovascular disease prevention programs in every state and U.S. territory. These recent mandates create a need and responsibility to formulate a long-range strategy to guide the public health community in preventing heart disease and stroke. Accordingly, in December 2001, CDC initiated a planning process that included an intensive series of expert consultations as the basis for developing this *Action Plan*.

Heart Disease and Stroke: Scope, Burden, Disparities, and a Forecast

The Scope of "Heart Disease and Stroke"

Disorders of the circulation that affect the heart, brain, and other organs may be described in various terms, sometimes with specific technical meaning.[1,3] For clarity, the most important terms used in this plan are defined either in the text or in the glossary (see Appendix A). Some of the more common terms are defined in this section.

"Heart disease and stroke" refers to the two major classes of circulatory conditions that are the main focus of the *Action Plan*. This usage, which was chosen for the title of the plan, corresponds with the terminology of Chapter 12, Heart Disease and Stroke of *Healthy People 2010*.[2] "Heart disease" most often refers to coronary heart disease (including heart attack and other effects of restricted blood flow through the arteries that supply the heart muscle) or to heart failure. Other times, this term refers to several conditions or all diseases affecting the heart (e.g., "heart disease deaths"). "Stroke" refers to a sudden impairment of brain function, sometimes termed "brain attack," that results from interruption of circulation to one or another part of the brain following either occlusion or hemorrhage of an artery supplying that area.

"Cardiovascular health" (CVH) refers broadly to a combination of favorable health habits and conditions that protects against the development of cardiovascular diseases. "CVH promotion" is support and dissemination of these favorable habits and conditions. "Cardiovascular disease or diseases" (CVD), in turn, refers in principle to any or all of the many disorders that can affect the circulatory system. Here, CVD most often means coronary heart disease (CHD), heart failure, and stroke, taken together, which are the circulatory system disorders of the greatest public health concern in the United States today. However, CVD can also mean cerebrovascular disease, or disease of brain circulation. Throughout this plan, which is intended to address heart disease and stroke together, use of either CVH or CVD means both cardiovascular and cerebrovascular disease. More often, if less conveniently, the phrase "heart disease and stroke" means explicitly that both are included.

Heart disease and stroke are mainly consequences of atherosclerosis and high blood pressure (hypertension).[3] They are sometimes included in the broader category of atherosclerotic and hypertensive diseases (see The Knowledge Base for Intervention later in this section). Risk factors for heart disease and stroke have been well established for many years. Distinct from age, family history, and possible genetic determinants are modifiable risk factors that cause heart attacks and strokes, including high blood cholesterol, high blood pressure, smoking, and diabetes. Behaviors that contribute to development of risk factors, partly by causing obesity, include adverse dietary patterns and physical inactivity. Social and environmental conditions that may determine such behavioral patterns, in turn, include education and income, cultural influences, family and personal habits, and opportunities to make favorable choices. Policies—especially in the form of laws, regulations, standards, or guidelines—contribute to setting these and other social and environmental conditions. For example, dietary patterns result from the influences of food production policies, marketing practices, product availability, cost, convenience, knowledge, choices that affect health, and preferences that are often based on early-life habits. Because many aspects of behavior are clearly beyond the control of the individual, the scope of heart disease and stroke prevention, from the public health perspective, extends far beyond the individual or the patient. Thus, a comprehensive public health strategy for prevention must address the broader determinants of risk and disease burden as they affect both the population as a whole and particular groups of special concern, including those determinants that make healthier choices more likely.

The Nation's CVD Burden

The nation's CVD burden can be described in many ways. Examples include the number and rate of deaths by age, sex, race or ethnicity, or place of residence; the number and percentage of the population with a specific CVD condition or risk factor; and estimates of economic costs, including direct health care expenditures and loss of income from early death or disability. Several federal agencies contribute data on these aspects of the burden, including CDC and its National Center for Health Statistics and NIH's National Heart, Lung, and Blood Institute and National Institute of Neurological Disorders and Stroke. Table 1 illustrates several measures of the CVD burden in the U.S. population as reported by the American Heart Association on the basis of these data sources.[1]

The dominant change in CVD mortality in the United States in recent decades was a major decline in the annual rates of death for the population as a whole (i.e., age-adjusted death rates) for both CHD and stroke. These declines resulted in a substantial reduction in the numbers of deaths from these conditions that would have occurred for any particular age group (e.g., 45–54 years) under the previously higher rates. Despite these declines in rates, actual numbers of deaths from heart disease have changed little in 30 years and have actually increased within the past decade, especially for stroke.[1] This is mainly because more people are living longer, and rates are higher among successively older age groups.

As a consequence, heart disease remains the nation's leading cause of death.[1] Stroke is the third leading cause of death, and both conditions are major causes of adult disability. The decline in rates of coronary heart disease mortality slowed from -3.3% a year in the 1980s to -2.7% a year in the 1990s, and the decline in overall rates of stroke mortality slowed markedly in contrast to the 1970s and 1980s.[4] Meanwhile, the frequency of heart failure increased steadily during the last 25 years.[3] Peripheral arterial disease continues to be a major predictor of CVD death.[1,3] In addition, the previous favorable trends were not uniform among racial and ethnic groups. For example, heart disease rates declined more slowly among blacks than whites.[1] These shifting trends are consistent with forecasts of the global burden of CVD over the next two decades and support the prediction that heart disease and stroke will persist as the leading causes of death and disability worldwide unless effective public health action is taken to prevent them.[5,6]

Two other points should be emphasized. First, sudden deaths from coronary heart disease that occur without hospitalization or in the absence of any previous medical history of coronary heart disease

Table 1. Selected indicators of the cardiovascular disease (CVD) burden, United States

Number of Deaths in 2000

2,600 CVD deaths occur every day—that's one every 33 seconds.

150,000 CVD deaths occur each year among people younger than age 65.

250,000 coronary heart disease (CHD) deaths occur each year without hospitalization.

50% of men and 63% of women who suffered a sudden CHD death lacked any previous CHD history.

40,429 deaths occurred in 2000 from peripheral vascular disease, aortic aneurysm, and other diseases of the arteries.

During 1990–2000, the number of CVD deaths increased 2.5%, although the death rate decreased 17.0%.

Survivors in 2000

450,000 people had survived a first heart attack for more than 1 year.

450,000 people had survived with heart failure for more than 1 year.

375,000 people had survived a first stroke for more than 1 year.

Prevalence in 2000

12.9 million people were living with coronary heart disease.

4.9 million people were living with heart failure.

4.7 million people were living with stroke.

Risk Factors in 2000

105 million people had high total cholesterol ($\geq$200 mg/dl).

50 million people had high blood pressure (systolic $\geq$140 mm Hg, diastolic $\geq$90 mm Hg) or were taking antihypertensive medication.

Nearly 48.7 million people age $\geq$18 were current smokers.

More than 44 million people were obese (body mass index $\geq$30.0 kg/m^2).

10.9 million people had physician-diagnosed diabetes.

Projected Costs in 2003

$209.3 billion in direct costs and $142.5 billion in indirect costs, for a total of $351.8 billion.

Note: Death rates and prevalence per 100,000 were age-adjusted to the 2000 U.S. standard population.
Source: Based on data compiled and reported by the American Heart Association. *Heart and Stroke Statistics—2003 Update.*

(250,000 each year) make the strongest case for prevention.[1] For some victims, no opportunity exists for treatment because their death is the first sign of CVD. Second, the annual cost of CVD to the nation is projected to exceed $351 billion in 2003.[1] This total includes direct health care costs (for hospital and nursing home care, physicians and other professionals, drugs and other medical durables, and home health care) and indirect costs (due to lost productivity from disability and death). This cost substantially exceeds comparable costs for all cancers ($202 billion) and for human immunodeficiency virus (HIV) infections ($28.9 billion) reported for 2002.[1]

Such data confirm that the CVD epidemic is continuing in the United States and that it is a major component of our health care costs. Yet they do not convey the full impact of CVD. For example, cognitive impairment and dementia caused by underlying vascular disease of the brain (vascular cognitive impairment [VCI]) may occur in as many as 30% of stroke survivors, as well as in people without a clear history of stroke.[7] These observations also apply to people with or without Alzheimer's disease. Such findings suggest that VCI is part of the CVD spectrum and should be included in estimates of both the CVD burden and the potential health and economic impact of prevention. These factors reinforce concerns that the aging of the U.S. population will make CVD an even greater burden than previously estimated in the next two decades.

The CVD burden can also be expressed in the personal stories of how it affects people and their families. Just one example is the sudden death from heart attack in June 2002 of the St. Louis Cardinals' star pitcher, Darryl Kile. Kile was 33 years old and is survived by his widow and three young children.[8] This is a striking example of the increased number of victims of sudden cardiac death younger than age 35 in the past decade.[1] With an estimated 12.9 million Americans living with heart disease and 4.7 million living with stroke, many people can recount the impact on their lives of becoming a victim of CVD. For millions of others who did not survive their first encounter with heart disease or stroke, only the family members or friends left behind can tell their stories.

Disparities

Health disparities have long been a special concern in setting national objectives, and *Healthy People 2010* calls for the elimination of such disparities as one of its two overarching goals.[2] Disparities can exist among certain populations defined by sex, race or ethnicity, education or income, disability, place of residence, or sexual orientation. Sex-specific data are commonly available for CVD. In contrast to previous beliefs, CVD is clearly not an affliction primarily of men. In fact, it causes more deaths among women. In 2000, CVD was responsible for 505,661 deaths among U.S. women and 440,175 deaths among U.S. men. The higher numbers among women are partially due to the greater numbers of women in the oldest age groups, where CVD mortality is highest.[1]

Major disparities in the burden of heart disease and stroke and their risk factors among different racial and ethnic groups are widely recognized. However, relevant data for some groups are scant or nonexistent because data have not been collected to address this concern adequately. To improve data collection, the federal government has promulgated standards for classifying race and ethnicity in federal data systems.[9]

Researchers have also explored and published data on the geographic variations in the burden of heart disease death—by state and by county— for both women and men in the five major racial and ethnic categories.[10,11] These publications include information on local economic resources and medical care resources in the different areas examined. Data on the geographic variations in stroke deaths were published in 2003.[12]

Table 2 summarizes heart disease mortality differences by race and ethnicity in the United States. Table 3 presents similar data for stroke deaths for the most recent years available, 1999–2000.*[12] Both tables illustrate striking disparities in the excess mortality among blacks (for both women and men) compared with all other groups.

---

* In Tables 2 and 3, data for Hispanics are presented twice—once under the category of "Hispanic," which includes Hispanics of all racial identities (e.g., Hispanic blacks, Hispanic whites), and again under any of the four racial categories according to a person's racial identity. Consequently, data for the five groups are not mutually exclusive because "Hispanic" is considered a designation of ethnicity, not race.

Table 2. Heart disease death rates for people aged ≥35 years, United States, 1991–1995*

Sex	Race or Ethnicity				
	American Indian or Alaskan Native	Asian or Pacific Islander	Black	Hispanic	White
Women	259	221	553	265	388
Men	465	372	841	432	666

* Rates per 100,000 are age-adjusted using the 1970 U.S. standard population.
Source: CDC. References 10 and 11.

Disparities in other areas have been published in *Health, United States, 2002*, an annual report on national trends in health statistics.[13] This report also examines differences in health outcomes and risk factors for major racial and ethnic groups in the United States. Table 4 (page 20) presents examples of these disparities, some of which relate specifically to heart disease and stroke, whereas others relate to overall health. Several key points about health disparities among different groups are evident in this table. First, the extent to which data are lacking for major population groups is evident. Second, for populations with adequate data, disparities are striking—particularly among African Americans—in terms of years of life lost to death from heart disease and cerebrovascular disease, prevalence of hypertension and obesity (women only), and poverty. Other noteworthy points are the low values of several indicators for Asians (including Native Hawaiians and Other Pacific Islanders); the excess years of life lost because of deaths from cerebrovascular disease and diabetes among American Indians or Alaska Natives; and the high prevalence in the Hispanic or Latino population of poverty, lack of health coverage, and obesity. The table also indicates that a substantial proportion of these three minority groups live in poverty or without health care coverage.

Table 3. Stroke death rates for people aged ≥35 years, United States, 1991–1998*

Sex	Race or Ethnicity				
	American Indian or Alaskan Native	Asian or Pacific Islander	Black	Hispanic	White
Women	77	96	153	72	113
Men	80	118	182	88	121

* Rates per 100,000 are age-adjusted using the 2000 U.S. standard population.
Source: CDC. Reference 12.

Although other data sources are available for some of these populations, they suffer several limitations. Some of these were outlined in a 1999 report that illustrated the insufficiencies of data on Asian American and Pacific Islander populations.[14] These include a lack of data for subgroups with heterogeneous health characteristics, relatively small sample sizes, a lack of systematic data collection, a lack of longitudinal studies, a lack of population-based CVD data, and self-selection bias in sampling methods. Eliminating disparities requires adequate CVD data to establish the nature and extent of the disparities and to monitor changes. Clearly, data systems must be strengthened if disparities are to be addressed effectively. What we do know about existing disparities indicates that interventions must affect disadvantaged groups more than they do the population as a whole. The population-based health objectives for heart disease and stroke presented in *Healthy People 2010* that could be improved in the short term have targets that are predominantly based on the criterion "better than the best"—that is, all groups are expected to achieve a better

Table 4. Disparities in selected health indicators by race/ethnicity, United States

Heath Indicators	American Indian or Alaska Native	Asian*	Black or African American	Native Hawaiian or Other Pacific Islander	White, Non-Hispanic	Hispanic or Latino
Years of potential life lost before age 75[†] from heart disease[‡] (1999 data)	1238.9	617.5	2398.9	—[§]	1222.9	869.8
Years of potential life lost before age 75[†] from CVD[‖] (1999 data)	243.3	214.4	508.2	—	180.8	207.5
Years of potential life lost before age 75[†] from diabetes mellitus[¶] (1999 data)	41.4	84.6	402.5	—	155.6	214.2
Tobacco use (cigarettes) during the past month among persons aged >12 (2000 data)	42.3%	16.5%	23.3%	—	25.9%	20.7%
Hypertension** among men aged 20–74 (1988–1994 data)	—	—	36.4%	—	25.5%	25.9%
Hypertension among women aged 20–74[††] (1988–1994 data)	—	—	35.9%	—	19.7%	22.3%
Total cholesterol ≥240 mg/dl among men (1988–1994 data)	—	—	16.4%	—	19.1%	18.7%
Total cholesterol ≥240 mg/dl among women (1988–1994 data)	—	—	19.5%	—	20.7%	17.7%
Body mass index ≥30 kg/m^2 among men aged ≥20 (1988–1994 data)	—	—	21.1%	—	20.7%	24.4%
Body mass index ≥30 kg/m^2 among women[††] aged ≥20 (1988–1994 data)	—	—	39.0%	—	23.3%	36.1%
No health care coverage among persons aged <65 (2000 data)[‡‡]	38.2%	17.3%	20.0%	—	15.2%	35.4%
Poverty, all[§§] (2000 data)	—	10.7%	22.0%	—	7.5%	21.2%
Poverty, aged <18, female head, no spouse[‖‖] (2000 data)	—	32.3%	49.4%	—	27.9%	48.3%

* Includes data for Native Hawaiians or other Pacific Islanders except for tobacco use.

† Rates per 100,000 are age-adjusted using the 2000 U.S. standard population.

‡ Includes all heart disease deaths coded according to the *International Statistical Classification of Diseases and Related Health Problems (ICD-10)* (Geneva, Switzerland: World Health Organization; 1992).

§ Data do not meet the criteria for statistical reliability, data quality, or confidentiality.

‖ Includes all cerebrovascular disease deaths coded according to the *ICD-10*.

¶ Includes all diabetes deaths coded according to the *ICD-10*.

** Defined as a person having blood pressure ≥140/90 mm Hg or reporting current antihypertensive therapy.

†† Excludes pregnant women.

‡‡ Percentages are age-adjusted using the 2000 U.S. standard population.

§§ Defined as all persons living in a household with income below the poverty level.

‖‖ Defined as all related children aged <18 years living in a household with income below the poverty level and headed by a female with no spouse present.

Note: Data on hypertension, total cholesterol, and body mass index (BMI) that are labeled "Hispanic or Latino" are for the Mexican population. Data labeled as "Black or African American" are for non-Hispanic blacks. Percentages are age-adjusted using the 2000 U.S. standard population.

Sources: CDC, NCHS, National Vital Statistics System: estimates of years of potential life lost. Substance Abuse and Mental Health Services Administration, National Household Survey on Drug Abuse: estimates of tobacco use. CDC, NCHS, National Health and Nutrition Examination Survey: estimates of hypertension, total cholesterol, and body mass index. CDC, NCHS, National Health Interview Survey: estimates of no health care coverage. U.S. Bureau of the Census, Current Population Survey: poverty.

measure of health status by 2010 than that of the most favorable group at the baseline.[2] This implies that we should attain health improvements for all groups within the population, but that groups with poorer baseline status need to experience accelerated improvement, so that all groups will reach the same measures of better health by 2010. Attaining the targets for these objectives will require that the most effective programs, including those aimed at reducing the prevalence of CVD risk factors, reach the groups with the greatest CVD burden.

A Forecast

Over the next two decades, the number of Americans older than age 65 will increase dramatically, from approximately 34.7 million in 2000 to more than 53.2 million in 2020.[15] By 2020, a total of 16.5% of Americans will be aged 65 or older, compared with 12.6% in 2000—an increase of nearly one-third. Proportions of minorities in the overall population are expected to increase from 12.9% to 14.0% for blacks, 4.1% to 6.1% for Asians, 0.9% to 1.0% for American Indians, and 11.4% to 16.3% for Hispanics. Heart disease deaths are projected to increase sharply between 2010 and 2030, and the population of heart disease survivors is expected to grow at a much faster rate than the U.S. population as a whole. Marked increases in numbers of stroke deaths are also predicted.[16] These changes together will constitute a major increase in the nation's CVD burden, accompanied by increasing demands for related health care services, as well as increases in health care expenditures; lost income and productivity; and prevalence of disease, disability, and dependency. This forecast suggests that instead of increasing quality and years of healthy life, we may lose ground. Moreover, if recent trends continue, disparities may widen rather than be eliminated.[4] The need for prevention has never been as great as it is today.

Myths and Misconceptions

Although data show us the hard facts, the disease burden also can be expressed in more visual ways to dramatize its magnitude. For example, the number of annual deaths from heart attacks alone exceeds the number of deaths that would occur if two fully occupied 747 aircraft crashed every day of the year with no survivors. Yet, CVD has not aroused a level of public concern commensurate with its relative importance.[1] Why?

Among the reasons are several myths or misconceptions about heart disease and stroke that must be addressed as this plan gains the needed support of the public and policy makers. These include the beliefs that heart attacks only affect the elderly, that heart attack death is quick and easy ("the best way to go"), that a heart attack can be "fixed" with modern medical and surgical technology, and that heart attacks and strokes occur when "your time has come."

The truth is very different. Of the 945,836 people who died of CVD in 2000, 32% were younger than age 75.[1] Currently, the average expected age at death in the United States is 76.9 years.[17] As noted previously,

250,000 coronary heart disease deaths occur each year without the victim reaching a hospital. For one-half to two-thirds of those who die suddenly of CHD, there was no previous recognition of the disease.[1] Many people who died under these conditions had no opportunity for treatment and could only have been saved by preventive measures that reach the population as a whole. The more common outcome, however, is to survive for days, weeks, months, or years. Those who survive may experience disability, job loss, or dependency, often with long-term consequences. Survivors also have a greatly increased risk of having another heart attack or stroke. Modern medicine and surgery can offer great benefit to those who survive long enough to receive treatment, but are no help to those who die suddenly following their first CVD event. There is no complete "cure" once a heart attack or stroke has occurred, as survivors continue to be at increased risk for another attack.[1] Finally, "your time" has not yet come if readily available preventive measures can still increase quality and years of healthy life.

These and other myths about heart disease and stroke must be dispelled through effective communication and education. They are significant barriers to understanding the urgency of the CVD epidemic and the potential for preventing these conditions.

The Knowledge Base for Intervention

The CVD epidemic in the United States and other Western industrialized countries was first recognized around the middle of the twentieth century.[3] In response, extensive research programs involving laboratory, clinical, and population-based investigations were undertaken to identify the causes and the means of preventing coronary heart disease and stroke. The result of this research has been a major growth in knowledge and understanding of the causes of CVD, especially because of the work of NIH and the American Heart Association.

Statistical research has shown that death rates from heart disease and stroke vary among populations and over only a few years' time in ways that cannot be explained by differences or changes in genetic factors. Such findings demonstrate clearly that environmental factors, in the broadest sense, play a major role in the occurrence of heart disease and stroke and can do so over a relatively short term. Thus, controlling these factors offers opportunities for prevention. Major epidemiologic studies revealed that incidence rates (measures of the occurrence of new cases of CVD, whether fatal or not) could be predicted by blood cholesterol level, blood pressure level, smoking, diabetes, and certain other potentially modifiable characteristics. These characteristics, recognized as "risk factors" since the 1960s, were ultimately established as the major causes of CVD.

How do these factors cause CVD? The principal pathway to a heart attack or stroke is through the gradual, years-long development of atherosclerosis and high blood pressure. Atherosclerosis is a disease of the medium-sized and larger arteries, such as those that supply the heart (the coronary arteries), the brain (the carotid and cerebral arteries), and the lower extremities (the peripheral arteries), as well as the aorta. Atherosclerosis consists of concentrated areas of mushy material (atheromas) within the arterial wall that are often encrusted or hardened (sclerosed) by deposited calcium. The resulting abnormality is a plaque that weakens the arterial wall and may intrude into the lumen or channel of the artery to limit blood flow or obstruct it completely. A plaque may suddenly rupture, leading to blockage of the artery and precipitating a heart attack or stroke.

High blood pressure (or hypertension) also can cause heart disease or stroke by exacerbating the effects of other risk factors in accelerating progression of atherosclerosis by placing a continuous, excess workload on the heart (hypertensive heart disease). It can also cause a cerebral artery to rupture (cerebral hemorrhage).

Atherosclerosis begins to develop in childhood and progresses into the adult years, under strong influence of the risk factors noted previously. Autopsy studies of young American men who died in the Korean War and in Vietnam confirmed that people in their 20s can have moderate and sometimes severe atherosclerosis despite a lack of any medical history to suggest it.[18,19] More recent studies of children, adolescents, and young adults (younger than 35) have demonstrated the close link of blood cholesterol level, blood pressure level, smoking, and obesity with the extent and severity of atherosclerosis among people well below age 20.[20,21] High blood pressure also develops progressively throughout life, undergoing major increases in adolescence and late adulthood. These findings underscore the opportunities for preventing CVD during childhood and adolescence, as well as the lifelong importance of prevention.

Establishing a way to prevent risk factors requires knowledge about the risk factors themselves. That is, can they be changed? Can heart attacks and strokes be prevented as a result? How prevalent are these risk factors? If their frequency is reduced in the population as a whole, what will the impact be on rates of heart disease and stroke nationwide? An impressive body of evidence amassed over the last 30 years has established that blood cholesterol levels, blood pressure levels, and smoking habits can be modified and that diabetes can be prevented and controlled by behavioral change as well as by medication, all with favorable impact on CVD risk. Population studies have monitored the continuing high prevalence of these risk factors in the United States since the early 1960s.

In the mid-1980s, researchers projected how the CVD burden would be affected if the major risk factors were reduced.[22] These projections suggested that CVD death rates could be reduced by 70% by reducing the population's mean level of blood cholesterol to 190 mg/dl and the mean level of diastolic blood pressure to 80 mm Hg. Because this estimate did not consider the added impact of reducing the prevalence of smoking, it probably underestimated how much CVD death rates could be reduced. Current estimates indicate that these major risk factors account for 75% of the difference in risk for CHD within populations.[23] If these projections were systematically updated, we could estimate how much the CVD burden might be reduced over the next two decades. This estimate might be substantially greater than the *Healthy People 2010* target of reducing heart disease and stroke deaths by 20%. As indicated previously, a greater reduction is needed if the projected increase in CVD burden is to be offset.

Finland's experiences during 1970–1990 are a good example of the healthy changes that can be achieved by reducing major risk factors for heart disease.[24] Improvements in blood cholesterol levels, blood pressure levels, and smoking rates for both women and men closely predicted the actual declines in heart disease deaths that were observed over 20 years. Deaths declined more than 60% for women and more than 50% for men. Although community intervention studies in the United States also have demonstrated positive changes, these interventions have generally lacked the intensity and duration (i.e., the "preventive dose") needed to demonstrate that they actually reduced CVD deaths beyond the influence of favorable changes taking place in society at large.[25]

What knowledge constitutes a sufficient basis for public health action? Both formal research and relevant practical experience are important. Like evidence-based medicine, evidence-based public health needs established criteria for systematically evaluating available evidence. Continuous evaluation can guide current and future programs and advance policies as new knowledge is acquired.

In contrast to evidence-based medicine, evidence-based public health depends on different types of evidence. For example, randomized controlled trials are considered essential to evidence-based medicine but are often lacking in the public health arena. On the other hand, population-based observations that are often unavailable in clinical decision making are included in the evidence base for public health decisions. The context of public health practice is the world at large, where many influences on health are continually at play. Therefore, the central question for evidence-based public health is not whether to take a particular action or no action, but whether the status quo, with its prevailing influences on the population's health, is best. By asking what evidence supports the status quo, as well as what supports a proposed alternative policy or program, evidence-based public health can help establish the relative merits of proposed interventions.

Clearly, the CVD burden of this nation will not improve under the status quo. We have the knowledge needed to launch a comprehensive public health strategy to change this situation. In fact, only by putting current knowledge into action now can we strengthen the body of knowledge substantially, as new and expanded programs and policy frameworks are implemented and rigorously evaluated.

Evolution of Prevention Policy

As our knowledge about CVD has grown during the past half-century, our policies for preventing heart disease and stroke have also advanced.[3] The first recommendations appeared in 1959 in *A Statement on*

Arteriosclerosis: Main Cause of "Heart Attacks" and "Strokes," which was signed by five past presidents of the American Heart Association.[26] Citing studies published in the 1950s, this report identified most of the same risk factors discussed here as the focus for preventive measures to be taken by patients and their physicians.

A wealth of recommendations has appeared subsequently. For example, the 1972 report from the Inter-Society Commission for Heart Disease Resources, *Primary Prevention of the Atherosclerotic Diseases*, recommended "a strategy of primary prevention of premature atherosclerotic diseases be adopted as long-term national policy for the United States and to implement this strategy that adequate resources of money and manpower be committed to accomplish: changes in diet to prevent or control hyperlipidemia, obesity, hypertension and diabetes; elimination of cigarette smoking; [and] pharmacologic control of elevated blood pressure."[27]

The Cardiovascular Disease Unit of the World Health Organization and the International Heart Health Conferences also have issued recommendations, usually addressing international and global concerns.[3,28] Recommendations have been published by the American Heart Association/American Stroke Association, the American College of Cardiology, and the National Heart, Lung, and Blood Institute, including clinical practice guidelines for detecting and treating risk factors and preventing heart disease and stroke.[3]

In 1994, an important predecessor to the present plan was published by the CVD Plan Steering Committee,* *Preventing Death and Disability from Cardiovascular Diseases: A State-Based Plan for Action*.[29] This document was a call to the states to expand their capacity and obtain additional resources so they could develop the infrastructure needed to achieve the year 2000 objectives for CVD prevention and control. By outlining basic functions for CVD programs and strategies for building capacity, this report contributed directly to implementation of CDC's state heart disease and stroke prevention program in 1998. It also indicated the value of partnership and collaborative in producing a policy document with broad support, based on the contributions of participating members.

In this extensive body of policy documents, what is advised for preventing heart disease and stroke? Two main approaches have been recommended—interventions addressing individuals and interventions addressing whole populations.[30] The individual or "high-risk" approach centers either on people with CVD risk factors but no evident disease or on those with CVD, including survivors of CVD events. For people with risk factors but no recognized disease, "primary prevention" is intended to prevent a first heart attack or stroke by detecting and treating risk factors. For people with known CVD, "secondary prevention" is

---

* Members represented the American Heart Association/American Stroke Association, the Association of State and Territorial Directors of Health Promotion and Public Health Education, the Association of State and Territorial Public Health Nutrition Directors, CDC, the Chronic Disease Directors, and the National Heart, Lung, and Blood Institute.

intended to reduce the risk for subsequent heart attacks or strokes by treating CVD and the risk factors. Both aspects focus on individual risk. The "population-wide" approach, which focuses on a whole population or community, recognizes that the excess risk for heart disease and stroke is widely distributed in the population, with most victims having moderate, rather than extreme, risk. Therefore, even modest change in average risk in the whole population, achievable through means such as public education, can markedly reduce the risk for CVD events.

A third approach aims to prevent CVD risk factors in the first place. Sometimes called "primordial prevention," this plan uses the term "CVH promotion."[31] This approach is most widely applicable in populations where social and economic development has yet to progress to the point of fostering epidemic occurrence of the major risk factors. CVH promotion also encompasses interventions aimed at individuals at any age who have not yet developed treatable levels of CVD risk factors because the interventions occur before the risk factors begin to cause or accelerate atherosclerosis. Such intervention should occur in childhood or even, as recent research suggests, during gestation (to improve the fetal environment).[32] These interventions should continue throughout adulthood to prevent risk factors from ever developing.

Despite the many policy recommendations made since the 1950s, practice has lagged far behind. Assessments in recent years have consistently shown that doctors and patients have not adhered well to treatment guidelines for secondary prevention.[33] Although well-supported and detailed policies for preventing heart disease and stroke have long been available, the actions recommended in these policies have, to a large degree, not been followed. Action is needed to support their effective implementation.

Healthy People 2010 Goals and Objectives

Published in January 2000, *Healthy People 2010* is the latest in a series of documents initiated in 1979 to present national health objectives.[2] This new volume makes an important advance over *Healthy People 2000* in presenting a goal and related objectives for preventing heart disease and stroke. The Healthy People 2010 Heart and Stroke Partnership* divided this goal into four separate goals based on the different intervention approaches that would be needed to achieve them. These four goals are prevention of risk factors, detection and treatment of risk factors, early identification and treatment of heart attacks and strokes, and prevention of recurrent cardiovascular events. Objectives outline specific measures of progress that should be attained by the year 2010. A total of 16 objectives specifically address coronary heart disease, heart

---

* Current partners include the American Heart Association/American Stroke Association; National Center for Chronic Disease Prevention and Health Promotion (NCCDPHP), CDC; Centers for Medicare & Medicaid Services; Indian Health Service; National Heart, Lung, and Blood Institute and National Institute of Neurological Disorders and Stroke, NIH; and Office of Disease Prevention and Health Promotion, Office of Public Health and Science, U.S. Department of Health and Human Services.

failure, stroke, blood pressure, and total blood cholesterol levels. In addition, 48 related objectives address chronic kidney disease, diabetes, nutrition and overweight, physical activity and fitness, tobacco use, access to quality health services, and public health infrastructure. Several other objectives relate indirectly to CVH. All of the related objectives are tabulated in Appendix B.

When the 2010 goal and its objectives were adopted, CDC was designated to join NIH as the co-lead federal health agency responsible for heart disease and stroke prevention. CDC and NIH share responsibility "for undertaking activities to move the nation toward achieving the year 2010 goals and for reporting progress . . . over the course of the decade."[2] The activities of these two co-lead agencies in heart disease and stroke prevention are highlighted in Appendix C. Publishing these goals and objectives alone will not assure that they are attained. When progress toward meeting the *Healthy People 2000* objectives was reviewed, three of the 17 objectives were met, some progress had been made for another 12 objectives, and health status had worsened for the remaining two.[34] Among the 9 objectives for which positive percentage changes could be calculated, only 5 reached more than 50% of the target.

Unless we make substantial progress toward meeting the 2010 goal for preventing heart disease and stroke, we will see increasing numbers of people with CVD risk factors, increasing numbers of first and recurrent heart attack and stroke victims, and increasing numbers of people who die of CVD. Further, costs will increase because of the larger numbers of people needing CVD treatment and the higher cost for each CVD event (if the trend of increasing costs for health services continues as expected). In contrast, success in meeting this goal can reverse the unfavorable trends of the past decade. We must build on the promise of knowledge and experience that awaits widespread translation into public health practice.

The Present Opportunity

To be effective, public health action must have a solid knowledge base that is built on science and practical experience and sound policies that are founded on this knowledge. Over the past 30 years, such support for heart disease and stroke prevention has been greatly strengthened. But this support has not been sufficient to establish and sustain the needed public health effort. Until the early 1970s, the Bureau of State Services in the former U.S. Department of Health, Education, and Welfare supported state health departments through its Heart Disease and Stroke Control Program, but that program was discontinued. And although the Inter-Society Commission on Heart Disease Resources called for a national commitment to prevent atherosclerosis in the early 1970s, public health efforts to address these problems have remained too limited to offer the full potential benefit of existing knowledge.[27]

What is different now from those early transient efforts? What new and unprecedented opportunities exist for heart disease and stroke prevention? This *Action Plan* describes the current opportunities for action and the potential for success in the immediate future. Recent trends in the CVD burden in the United States and projections of the continuing predominance of heart disease and stroke as causes of death and disability worldwide have motivated concerned health professionals to consider a new level of concerted action to prevent CVD.[4,5] Clearly, treating victims of heart disease and stroke cannot alone solve the problem. Prevention is preferable in principle and necessary as a matter of national policy if we are to attain our goals of increasing quality and years of healthy life and eliminating health disparities. This perspective has recently been strongly reinforced by *Steps to a HealthierUS*, a bold new initiative by Secretary of Health and Human Services Tommy G. Thompson. The *Steps* initiative is designed to address this nation's health care crisis and the need to prevent the chronic diseases and conditions, including heart disease and stroke, that represent 75% of our health care expenditures. The Secretary's initiative is a response to President George W. Bush's *HealthierUS* initiative, which directs key departments of the federal government to develop plans to better promote fitness and health for all Americans.

To implement *Steps to a HealthierUS*, the U.S. Department of Health and Human Services (HHS) is marshalling all available resources within the department and calling on other federal agencies and the private sector (e.g., the fast food and soft drink industries) to take steps to improve our nation's health. At the personal level, all Americans are challenged to take the first step by walking 30 minutes a day. At the societal level, policy makers are asked to take their first step by embracing prevention as the long-term solution for our health care crisis. The *Steps* initiative thus constitutes a significant impetus toward prevention, which is strongly supported by this *Action Plan*.

The breadth of the 2010 goal for preventing heart disease and stroke calls attention to the wide range of opportunities for intervention— both to prevent CVD through primary and secondary prevention and to promote CVH. This goal also underscores the increased role for public health agencies, including CDC. As population-wide approaches become more common, the skills and resources of public health agencies at all levels of government will be increasingly called upon.

In recent years, it has also been realized that effective, concerted action requires partnerships with familiar organizations and agencies, as well as with nontraditional partners with distinct perspectives and contributions. As a result, new alliances are being formed, and new ideas, expertise, and resources are being shared. The Healthy People 2010 Heart and Stroke Partnership is a good example of this type of partnership, which can potentially include partners within and beyond the health sector. Already, channels of communication have been opened that will help identify common areas of interest and opportunities for synergy among these national organizations and agencies. Additional agreements between federal agencies and other organizations further illustrate the development of key partnerships in CVH.

Recent advances in knowledge heighten confidence that public health intervention can improve on our CVD forecast for the next two decades. For example, researchers demonstrated that high blood pressure can be prevented with dietary interventions.[35] We now know that diabetes can be prevented or delayed with dietary and physical activity interventions.[36] And recent findings strongly suggest that by preventing CVD risk factors from emerging in adolescence and early adulthood, we can expect to prevent atherosclerosis later in life.[20] Evidence that blood cholesterol and blood pressure levels are improving in the population reinforce the belief that positive changes are occurring and can be accelerated, even while adverse changes (e.g., the obesity and diabetes epidemics) call for more innovative approaches to reverse these alarming trends.[37,38]

The health of this nation is the central focus of the *Action Plan*, but not to the exclusion of concern for the global dimensions of the burden of heart disease and stroke and recognition of the potential value of international collaboration in their prevention. The Global Burden of Disease Study, cited earlier, stated that heart disease and stroke were the foremost causes of death throughout the world in 1990 and projected that they will remain so in 2020.[5] In its 1999 report, *Impending Global Pandemic of Cardiovascular Diseases*, the World Heart Federation provides extensive documentation of this epidemic, as well as resources and strategies by which to address it.[39]

In the same year, the Director-General of the World Health Organization presented a report titled, *Global Strategy for the Prevention and Control of Noncommunicable Diseases*, which noted that, "Four of the most prominent noncommunicable diseases—cardiovascular disease, cancer, chronic obstructive pulmonary diseases and diabetes—are linked by common preventable risk factors related to lifestyle. These factors are tobacco use, unhealthy diet and physical inactivity . . . Intervention at the level of the family and community is essential for prevention because the causal risk factors are deeply entrenched in the social and cultural framework of the society. Addressing the major risk factors should be given the highest priority in the global strategy for the prevention and control of noncommunicable diseases."[40]

A major contribution toward this end is *The World Health Report 2002: Reducing Risks, Promoting Healthy Life*.[6] This report presents an extensive analysis of the major risk factors and the potential impact of their prevention and control on the burden of cardiovascular and other chronic diseases throughout the world. The report notes, "In order to protect people—and help them protect themselves—governments need to be able to assess risks and choose the most cost-effective and affordable interventions to prevent risks from occurring."[6] Significant advances in approaches and methods for such an assessment are offered by that report.

Does this nation have a role in the global arena of heart disease and stroke prevention? Addressing this question, the Institute of Medicine's 1997 report, *America's Vital Interest in Global Health*, concluded that ". . . the United States should build on its strengths and seize the unprecedented opportunities to work with its international partners to improve health worldwide."[41] Proposed action areas included biomedical research and development, education and training in the health sciences, and effective international cooperation. An underlying premise of the report was that "global health problems affect all peoples in all countries and transcend national boundaries, levels of development, and political systems."[41] A sequel to this report, *Control of Cardiovascular Diseases in Developing Countries: Research, Development, and Institutional Strengthening*, appeared in 1998 and recommended specific steps to be taken to assess the burden, develop intervention plans, and take effective action country by country.[42] At the same time, it was noted that, "Many organizations and programs are engaged in activities relevant to CVD prevention and control. The impact of their work can be enhanced, and duplication avoided, by effective exchange of information on CVD activities."[42]

These recent reports, which have documented the global problem of CVD and the growing recognition of its worldwide importance, strongly suggest that this nation does have a role in the global arena of heart disease and stroke prevention. This role includes providing information from our own experiences to support the work of others and gaining from their growing knowledge and experience in return. Another basis for this view stems from the position of HHS, which is conducting and supporting programs to advance global health issues, including policy development, public health infrastructure strengthening, scientific research and research training, and tobacco control (see www.hhs.gov/news/press/2002pres/global.html). The recommendations of this *Action Plan* for engaging in regional and global partnerships for heart disease and stroke prevention are in full accord with this view.

The challenging circumstances we face today, in combination with significant advances in research, provide strong justification for developing a public health action plan to prevent heart disease and stroke. In response, this *Action Plan* has been developed. If effectively implemented, this plan can arrest or reverse the epidemic of heart disease and stroke in the United States and contribute substantially to preventing these conditions throughout the world.

References

1. American Heart Association. *2003 Heart and Stroke Statistics—2003 Update*. Dallas, TX: American Heart Association; 2003.

2. US Department of Health and Human Services. *Healthy People 2010: Understanding and Improving Health and Objectives for Improving Health*. 2nd ed. Vol 1. Washington, DC: US Government Printing Office; November 2000.

3. Labarthe DR. *Epidemiology and Prevention of Cardiovascular Diseases: A Global Challenge*. Gaithersburg, MD: Aspen Publishers; 1998.

4. Cooper R, Cutler J, Desvigne-Nickens P, et al. Trends and Disparities in Coronary Heart Disease, Stroke, and Other Cardiovascular Diseases in the United States. Findings of the National Conference on Cardiovascular Disease Prevention. *Circulation* 2000;102:3137–47.

5.   Murray CJL, Lopez A. Alternative Projections of Mortality and Disability by Cause 1990–2020: Global Burden of Disease Study. *Lancet* 1997;349: 1498–1504.

6.   World Health Organization. *The World Health Report 2002: Reducing Risks, Promoting Healthy Life.* Geneva: World Health Organization; 2002.

7.   Gorelick PB. Prevention. In: Erkinjuntti T, Gauthier S, editors. *Vascular Cognitive Impairment.* London: Martin Dunitz LTD; 2002:571–86.

8.   The Associated Press. Playing Through the Pain. *Atlanta Journal Constitution* 2002 June 24;Sect. D:1.

9.   Office of Management and Budget. *Standards for the Classification of Federal Data on Race and Ethnicity.* Washington, DC: Executive Office of the President, Office of Management and Budget; 1994. Available at www.whitehouse.gov/omb/fedreg/notice_15.html.

10.   Casper ML, Barnett E, Halverson JA, et al. *Women and Heart Disease: An Atlas of Racial and Ethnic Disparities in Mortality. Second Edition.* Morgantown, WV: Office for Social Environment and Health Research; 2000.

11.   Barnett E, Casper ML, Halverson JA, et al. *Men and Heart Disease: An Atlas of Racial and Ethnic Disparities in Mortality. First Edition.* Morgantown, WV: Office for Social Environment and Health Research; 2001.

12.   Casper ML, Barnett E, Williams GI Jr, et al. *Atlas of Stroke Mortality: Racial, Ethnic, and Geographic Disparities in the United States.* Atlanta, GA: US Department of Health and Human Services, Centers for Disease Control and Prevention; January 2003.

13.   Centers for Disease Control and Prevention. *Health, United States, 2002. With Chartbook on Trends in the Health of Americans.* Hyattsville, MD: US Department of Health and Human Services, Centers for Disease Control and Prevention; 2002. DHHS publication no. 1232.

14.   Asian & Pacific Islander American Health Forum. *A Public Health Action Plan. Eliminating Racial and Ethnic Disparities in Cardiovascular Health: Improving the Cardiovascular Health of Asian American and Pacific Islander Populations in the United States.* San Francisco, CA: Asian & Pacific Islander American Health Forum; 1999.

15.   Foot DK, Lewis RP, Pearson TA, Beller GA. Demographics and Cardiology, 1950–2050. *Journal of the American College of Cardiology* 2000;35:(No. 5 Suppl B):66B–80B.

16.   Howard G, Howard VJ. Stroke Incidence, Mortality, and Prevalence. In: Gorelick PB, Alter M, editors. *The Prevention of Stroke.* New York, NY: The Parthenon Publishing Group; 2002:1–10.

17.   Minino AM, Arias E, Kochanek KD, Murphy SL, Smith BL. Deaths: Final Data for 2000. Hyattsville, MD: US Department of Health and Human Services, Centers for Disease Control and Prevention; 2002. (*National Vital Statistics Reports*, vol 50, no. 15).

18.   Enos WF, Holmes RH, Beyer J. Coronary Disease Among United States Soldiers Killed in Action in Korea. *JAMA* 1953;152:1090–3.

19.   McNamara JJ, Molot MA, Stremple JF, Cutting RT. Coronary Artery Disease in Combat Casualties in Vietnam. *JAMA* 1971;216:1185–7.

20.   Berenson GS, Wattigney WA, Tracy RE, et al. Atherosclerosis of the Aorta and Coronary Arteries and Cardiovascular Risk Factors in Persons Ages 6 to 30 Years and Studied at Necropsy (the Bogalusa Heart Study). *American Journal of Cardiology* 1992;70:851–8.

21.   Pathobiological Determinants of Atherosclerosis in Youth (PDAY) Research Group. Relationship of Atherosclerosis in Young Men to Serum Lipoprotein Cholesterol Concentrations and Smoking. *JAMA* 1990;264:3018–24.

22.   Kottke TE, Puska P, Salonen JT, Tuomilehto J, Nissinen A. Projected Effects of High-Risk Versus Population-Based Prevention Strategies in Coronary Heart Disease. *American Journal of Epidemiology* 1984;121:697–704.

23.   Magnus P, Beaglehole R. The Real Contribution of the Major Risk Factors to the Coronary Epidemics: Time to End the "Only 50%" Myth. *Archives of Internal Medicine* 2001;161:2657–60.

24. Puska P, Tuomilehto J, Nissinen A, Vartiainen E, editors. *The North Karelia Project: 20 Year Results and Experiences.* Finland: National Public Health Institute (KTL); 1995.

25. O'Connor B, Cameron R, Farquharson J, et al. Marketing the Heart Health Vision: Delivering the "Preventive Dose." Ottawa, Canada: WHO Collaborating Centre for Policy Development in the Prevention of Noncommunicable Disease; 2000.

26. White PD, Wright IS, Sprague HB, et al. *A Statement on Arteriosclerosis: Main Cause of "Heart Attacks" and "Strokes."* New York, NY: National Health Education Committee, Inc.; 1959.

27. Atherosclerosis Study Group (Stamler J, chair), Epidemiology Study Group (Lilienfeld A, chair). Primary Prevention of the Atherosclerotic Diseases. In: Wright IS, Frederickson DT. *Cardiovascular Diseases. Guidelines for Prevention and Care.* Reports of the Inter-Society Commission for Heart Disease Resources. New York, NY: Inter-Society Commission for Heart Disease Resources; 1972:44.

28. Wilson E, Farquhar JW, O'Connor B, Harriman ME, McLean D, Pearson TA. *International Action On Cardiovascular Disease: A Platform For Success* (in press).

29. CVD Plan Steering Committee. *Preventing Death and Disability from Cardiovascular Diseases: A State-Based Plan for Action.* Washington, DC: Association of State and Territorial Health Officers; 1994.

30. Rose G. Strategy of Prevention: Lessons from Cardiovascular Disease. *BMJ* 1981;282:1847–51.

31. Strasser T. Reflections on Cardiovascular Diseases. *Interdisciplinary Science Reviews* 1978;3:225–30.

32. Barker DSP, editor. Fetal and Infant Origins of Adult Disease. London: *British Medical Journal*; 1992.

33. Pearson TA, McBride PE, Miller NH, Smith SC Jr. Task Force 8: Organization of Preventive Cardiology Service. *Journal of the American College of Cardiology* 1996;27:1039–47.

34. US Department of Health and Human Services. *Healthy People 2000 Final Review.* Washington, DC: US Department of Health and Human Services; 2001. DHHS publication no. 01-0256.

35. Sacks FM, Svetkey LP, Vollmer WM, et al. Effects on Blood Pressure of Reduced Dietary Sodium and the Dietary Approaches to Stop Hypertension (DASH) Diet. DASH-Sodium Collaborative Research Group. *New England Journal of Medicine* 2001;344:3–10.

36. Knowler WC, Barrett-Connor E, Fowler SE, et al and the Diabetes Prevention Program Research Group. Reduction in the Incidence of Type 2 Diabetes with Lifestyle Intervention or Metformin. *New England Journal of Medicine* 2002;346:393–403.

37. Goff DC Jr, Howard G, Russell GB, Labarthe DR. Birth Cohort Evidence of Primary Prevention of High Blood Pressure in the United States, 1887–1994. *Annals of Epidemiology* 2000;11:271–9.

38. Goff DC Jr, Labarthe DR, Howard G and Russell GB. Primary prevention of high blood cholesterol concentrations in the United States. *Archives of Internal Medicine* 2002;162:913–9.

39. Chockalingam A, Balaguer-Vintró I, editors. *Impending Global Pandemic of Cardiovascular Diseases.* Barcelona: Prous Science; 1999.

40. Brundtland GH. *Global Strategy for the Prevention and Control of Noncommunicable Diseases.* Geneva: World Health Organization; 1999:1.

41. Institute of Medicine. *America's Vital Interest in Global Health.* Washington, DC: National Academy Press; 1997:44, 46.

42. Institute of Medicine. *Control of Cardiovascular Diseases in Developing Countries: Research, Development, and Institutional Strengthening.* Washington, DC: National Academy Press; 1998:60.

SECTION 2.
A COMPREHENSIVE PUBLIC HEALTH STRATEGY AND THE FIVE ESSENTIAL COMPONENTS OF THE PLAN: A PLATFORM FOR ACTION

Summary

Section 2 presents a vision of cardiovascular health (CVH) that is achievable through a comprehensive public health strategy. Such a strategy will guide the needed action, from preventing heart disease and stroke among healthy people to treating and managing these conditions when prevention has failed. To develop the strategy, an action framework was developed that outlines the present reality, a vision of the future, and six broad intervention approaches that can help achieve this vision. These six approaches address the two overarching goals of *Healthy People 2010*, which are to increase quality and years of healthy life and eliminate health disparities, as well as the specific goal for preventing heart disease and stroke.

The action framework helps to distinguish two widely recognized aspects of intervention—health promotion and disease prevention—as they apply to heart disease and stroke. It also describes the nature and magnitude of the target population for each intervention approach. These descriptions illustrate a striking imbalance between the lack of investment in prevention—when risk is still low—and the massive expenditures for health care once recognized cardiovascular disease (CVD) has developed. A comprehensive public health strategy must address this imbalance.

The meaning of "public health" is central to the concept of a comprehensive public health strategy and is clearly stated in the 1988 Institute of Medicine report, *The Future of Public Health*. That report defined public health and its core functions and emphasized that state public health agencies have the primary responsibility for these functions. The report also described the potential roles of other parties, including health agencies at federal, state, and local (i.e., county/city) levels; health care providers; other partners in and outside the health sector; the public at large; and representatives of specific population groups or particular target settings.

To proceed from a comprehensive public health strategy to a practical plan of action requires that specific recommendations be developed and concrete action steps be proposed. Accordingly, recommendations and related action steps are presented in five essential areas that constitute the core of this plan.

Introduction: A Vision of Cardiovascular Health for America

A challenging vision of cardiovascular health for the United States is a nation whose residents are heart-healthy and stroke-free. Can we reach this vision from the present reality? What will the CVD burden be like in such a future? By what means can so radical a change be achieved? What roles will public health agencies and others need to play? What action areas must be addressed in developing appropriate recommendations?

To effectively address these questions, we must develop a framework for addressing the questions, understand the role and responsibilities of public health agencies, and define the major action areas so that the most pertinent issues can be identified and corresponding recommendations formulated.

A Framework for a Comprehensive Public Health Strategy

Developing a comprehensive public health strategy requires considering the full scope of a public health problem and the array of potential approaches to controlling it. It also requires recognizing the present reality and having a vision of the future that includes the most favorable conditions that can result from effective public health action. Bringing these four elements together in one action framework provides guidance and helps ensure that all relevant aspects are addressed. The framework developed for the *Action Plan* provides a useful point of reference for considering the recommendations and proposed action steps (see figure on inside back cover).

This framework is intended to represent the full scope of CVH in all its aspects, including the progressive development of CVD and the corresponding opportunities for CVH promotion and CVD prevention. It reflects the extensive research and practical experience of the past 50 years and more, which have provided a solid understanding of the causes of CVD and identified a wide range of opportunities for intervention. The framework also indicates where intervention approaches can be applied, through greatly expanded public health efforts, to advance from the present reality toward the vision of the future.

The Present Reality

The present reality of the burden of heart disease and stroke, especially in the United States, was documented in Section 1.[1,2] Underlying this burden are the long-term development of atherosclerosis and high blood pressure, conditions that are widely prevalent throughout our society. The causes begin with unfavorable social and environmental conditions that foster adverse behavioral patterns and result in a high prevalence of major risk factors. Inadequate measures for preventing, detecting, and controlling risk factors lead to first CVD events (e.g., heart attack, heart failure, stroke) from which many victims die suddenly, while others survive with a high risk for recurrence and often with disability. Many victims ultimately suffer fatal complications or cardiovascular decompensation months or years after the initial event.

A Vision of the Future

We envision a future when the epidemic of heart disease and stroke has been arrested and reversed. This future includes social and environmental conditions that are favorable to health, a predominance of health-promoting behaviors, a low prevalence of risk factors, fewer and less frequently fatal CVD events, rapid recovery of full functional capacity for victims who survive, and good quality of life thereafter until death from whatever cause. The critical question is, how do we move from the present reality to this vision of the future?

Intervention Approaches

The answer can be found in the six-fold array of intervention approaches available today. First, policy and environmental change addresses fundamental social and environmental conditions that operate early in CVD development; this approach can also influence later phases of the disease process (e.g., by improving accessibility, use, and quality of health care).[3] Second, behavioral change, especially population-wide, can reduce the effects of adverse social and environmental conditions. It can also reinforce the approaches that follow (e.g., by fostering community awareness and support for heart disease and stroke prevention). The third approach—detecting and controlling risk factors—has been a mainstay of CVD prevention and is needed continually once risk factors are present, to prevent both first and recurrent CVD events. (This approach comes too late in the process to prevent the risk factors themselves.) The fourth approach is emergency care and acute case management for those victims of first events who survive long enough to receive intervention. This approach continues to apply when survivors of previous acute CVD events experience recurrent ones. The fifth approach is rehabilitation, which should be applied following most acute events, and long-term management, which continues throughout the remainder of a victim's life until the sixth approach, end-of-life care, may be required.

Healthy People 2010 Goals

The action framework establishes a clear link between the proposed comprehensive public health strategy and *Healthy People 2010* goals.[4] Together, the six intervention approaches will help achieve the two overarching goals of *Healthy People 2010*, as well as the specific goal for preventing heart disease and stroke. The Healthy People 2010 Heart and Stroke Partnership divided this goal into four separate goals based on the different intervention approaches that would be needed to achieve them.

Target Population

Each intervention approach has the potential to affect millions of people in the United States.[1] The total U.S. population of 281 million people stands to benefit from policy and environmental change and population-wide behavioral change. The more than 100 million people with risk factors (e.g., high cholesterol, high blood pressure, smoking, obesity, diabetes) could benefit from effective risk factor detection and control. In addition, the hundreds of thousands of victims of first major CVD events each year can gain from acute or long-term case management and, potentially, from end-of-life care.

Interventions with the greatest impact on the population as a whole are those applied in the earliest phases of CVD development. To treat victims of heart disease, stroke, or other cardiovascular conditions is clearly to intervene late in the disease process. For those who die suddenly without warning, it is too late to have any benefit. Today, only a few cents per person per year are invested in the most far-reaching intervention approaches, whereas thousands of dollars per person per year are spent in efforts to treat established risk factors, rescue the victims of acute events, restore function and reduce risk for recurrent events among survivors, and provide end-of-life care. There is a need and opportunity to support a continuum of care, from the whole population to the individual victims of CVD, but we as a nation are not doing so. To attain our vision of the future and achieve the applicable goals of *Healthy People 2010*, a change in the balance of investment between early and late intervention is needed. A comprehensive public health strategy to prevent heart disease and stroke must aim for greatly increased application of the earliest intervention approaches, while working toward assurance that appropriate services of high quality will be accessible and used by all those who continue to need them. In the vision of the future, that need will be substantially reduced.

Finally, the action framework offers a clearer understanding of CVH promotion and CVD prevention, as these terms are defined and used in the *Action Plan* (see Section 1 and Appendix A). CVH promotion is intended to prevent risk factors (goal 1) and includes policy and environmental change and behavioral change, especially at the population level. CVD prevention applies to subsequent phases of CVD development and includes primary and secondary prevention. Primary prevention is intended to prevent first clinical events by detecting and treating risk factors (goal 2), whereas secondary prevention follows the first event and, for victims who survive, seeks to restore full functional capacity and reduce the risk of recurrence (goal 4). Goal 3, early detection and treatment of heart attacks and strokes, is part of CVD prevention and falls between primary and secondary prevention.

The Three Core Functions of Public Health

For many people, addressing the meaning of "public health" and clarifying its essential role in protecting society from such chronic diseases as heart disease and stroke may be helpful. The 1988 IOM report, *The Future of*

Public Health, was a critical assessment of the nation's public health system by the Committee for the Study of the Future of Public Health.[5] The findings of that report provide an important perspective on what will be needed for a successful public health strategy to prevent heart disease and stroke. The following excerpts illustrate this point.

- **A definition of public health:** *Public health is what we, as a society, do collectively to assure the conditions in which people can be healthy.*
- **A key barrier to public health action:** *Health officials have difficulty communicating a sense of urgency about the need to maintain current preventive efforts and to sustain the capability to meet future threats to the public's health.*
- **The report's overall appraisal:** . . . *this nation has lost sight of its public health goals and has allowed the system of public health activities to fall into disarray.*
- **The needed response:** *This report conveys an urgent message to the American people. Public health is a vital function that is in trouble. Immediate public concern and support are called for in order to fulfill society's interest in assuring the conditions in which people can be healthy.*

Especially relevant to the development of the *Action Plan* is the IOM report's formulation of the three core functions of public health: ". . . the core functions of public health agencies at all levels of government are assessment, policy development, and assurance." Assessment refers to the obligation of every public health agency to monitor the health status and needs of its community regularly and systematically. Policy development refers to the responsibility of every public health agency to develop comprehensive policies that are based on available knowledge and responsive to communities' health needs. Assurance is the guarantee of governments that agreed-upon, high-priority personal and community health services will be provided to every member of the community by qualified organizations.

Each of the recommendations in this plan is readily identifiable with one of these three core functions or addresses requirements for public health agencies to fulfill them. The recommendations also reflect many of the perceptions about the roles and relationships of public health agencies and other entities in the IOM report. Two points are especially relevant. First is the scope of participation needed to achieve public health goals. Private and voluntary organizations and individuals must join with government entities in actively contributing to the functions of public health. Second, state public health agencies have primary constitutional responsibility for public health functions. This premise is reflected in this plan's development and the expectation that these agencies must have a central role in implementing its recommendations.

In this respect, as in many others, the views of the five Expert Panels that helped develop the *Action Plan* closely matched those expressed in the 1988 report. They also reflected agreement with the conceptual framework described here. Subsequent to the work of the Expert Panels, two new IOM reports on the present and future of public health in the United States have been released, and both of them strongly reinforce the recommendations presented here.[6,7] The first, *Who Will Keep the Public Healthy?*, focuses on new requirements for educating health professionals for the 21st century. It presents an ecological model (i.e., "a model of health that emphasizes the linkages and relationships among multiple determinants affecting health") as the essential backdrop, both in concept and in practice, for addressing future health challenges. The framework guiding development of the *Action Plan* is such a model. Further, the newly formulated goals and objectives for educating health professionals closely mirror the recommendations for strengthening capacity of the public health workforce.

The second report, *The Future of the Public's Health in the 21st Century*, builds on the 1988 report. It emphasizes a broad view of the "public health system" that encompasses the governmental public health infrastructure as well as other potential partners, specifically the community, health care delivery system, employers and businesses, media, and academia. This report also explicitly embraces the vision of the nation's health expressed by *Healthy People 2010*: "healthy people in healthy communities." Topics addressed in the report include "adopting a focus on population health that includes multiple determinants of health; strengthening the public health infrastructure; building partnerships; developing systems of accountability; emphasizing evidence; and improving communication." The congruence between recommendations of the *Action Plan* and the IOM's recent reassessment of what is needed to strengthen the nation's public health system is striking.

Potential Roles of Partners

The *Action Plan* recognizes the necessary scope of participation in public health activities expressed in the 1988 IOM report and highlights the need for partnership, collaboration, and shared responsibility. Although state health agencies are primarily responsible for fulfilling the core functions of public health, the potential roles of private and voluntary organizations and individuals in public health activities are also important.[5] In anticipation of the involvement of various types of organizations and agencies, general descriptions of these roles are as follows:

- **Public health agencies** are responsible for leadership in convening all participating organizations and agencies to define and delineate tasks and to support the long-term implementation of this plan at national, state, and local levels. Agencies will participate in accordance with their particular missions, interests, and resources. Some are already involved through the Healthy People 2010 Heart and Stroke Partnership. State and local (i.e., county/city) health agencies and tribal organizations will help guide national implementation and take direct responsibility for action at their own levels.

- **Health care providers** are central to the provision of preventive services throughout the clinical phases of CVD. Addressing goals 2–4 of the Healthy People 2010 Heart and Stroke Partnership requires active collaboration with providers, third-party payers, and other relevant partners to assure access to and appropriate use of quality health services by those who need them.

- **Other health-sector partners** will help implement the plan at national, state, or local levels, as appropriate. Their roles include contributing to detailed implementation plans, raising public awareness, and supporting legislative and regulatory action to fulfill the plan's policy goals.

- **Non–health-sector partners** represent such areas as education, agriculture and food production, community development and planning, parks and recreation, transportation, and the media. These partners can contribute different perspectives, as well as additional resources, to help implement the plan and are clearly essential for success.

- **The public at large and representatives of specific groups or settings** are critical parties to public health action of any kind. Engaging these parties is also essential to the plan's implementation and success.

- **All interested parties and stakeholders** should be included in implementation, and mechanisms for their involvement must be established and maintained.

Five Essential Components of the *Action Plan*

The third requirement for a comprehensive public health strategy is defining the action areas in which recommendations are needed. An independent Expert Panel was convened to address each of five components considered essential to this plan—taking action, strengthening capacity, evaluating impact, advancing policy, and engaging in regional and global partnerships. Each component is best characterized by brief statements from the five panels, indicating their perspective on their charge and the theme of the resulting recommendations. The linkages of these five components form an integrated plan (see Figure 2 in Overview). Each panel's recommendations are presented in Section 3. Details of the planning process and the premises that guided each panel's work are outlined in Appendix D.

- **Taking action:** Putting present knowledge to work (Expert Panel A).

   Perspective: Acting now on what is already known must be the first priority. The greatest need is to implement the most promising policies and programs for heart disease and stroke prevention immediately and to the fullest extent feasible. Effective communication and innovative leadership, partnerships, and organizational arrangements are required.

   Theme: Federal, state, and local public health agencies urgently need explicit mandates and adequate resources to effectively implement policies and programs to prevent chronic diseases and to arrest and reverse the continuing national epidemic of heart disease and stroke.

- **Strengthening capacity:** Transforming the organization and structure of public health agencies and partnerships (Expert Panel B).

Perspective: Effective action to prevent heart disease and stroke requires transformation in how public health agencies are organized. Strengthening the competencies and resources of the public health workforce for the needed tasks and managing the development, maintenance, and dynamic growth of effective partnerships are necessary for this change.

Theme: Public health agencies must develop and maintain new capacities, including organizational arrangements and competencies for CVH promotion and CVD prevention. They also need networks of established and innovative partnerships to fulfill their mandates to prevent heart disease and stroke.

- **Evaluating impact:** Monitoring the disease burden, measuring progress, and communicating urgency (Expert Panel C).

Perspective: Action must be guided by 1) continuous, comprehensive assessment of all aspects of the public health burden of CVD; 2) identification of opportunities for effective intervention; and 3) prediction and evaluation of the impact of actions taken. At present, essential information for planning and evaluation is often unavailable for priority populations or the population as a whole. The needed data include key indicators of social and environmental conditions; patterns of behavior; incidence and prevalence of risk factors, as well as the status of their detection, treatment, and control; and incidence of first and recurrent CVD events, case fatality, hospitalization, mortality, disability, and survival. Data sources must be enhanced and used more effectively for assessment, policy development, and assurance at local, state, and national levels. Major gaps in data systems must be closed (e.g., by monitoring incidence of risk factors and events), workforce needs must be met (e.g., for data collection, analysis, interpretation, reporting, and dissemination), and new data sources must be established (e.g., to expand coverage of populations at high risk and establish a network of sentinel communities for comprehensive population-based monitoring and surveillance).

Theme: To guide and document progress toward national goals for heart disease and stroke prevention, public health agencies at all levels must establish and maintain substantially improved systems of data collection, analysis, and reporting. These systems must meet requirements for monitoring key *Healthy People 2010* leading health indicators, evaluating the impact and effectiveness of policies and programs, and communicating this information rapidly. All such systems must conform to the highest standards of data quality and reliability.

- **Advancing policy:** Defining the issues and finding the needed solutions (Expert Panel D).

  Perspective: The effectiveness of actions taken to prevent heart disease and stroke in coming years can increase as the foundation of evidence-based public health decision making is strengthened. A well-developed and continually updated agenda for CVD prevention research will support this growth. This research agenda must address critical policy issues through targeted investigations and scientific oversight; potential research settings, funding mechanisms, and evaluation plans require attention as well.

  For example, if atherosclerosis and high blood pressure (major causes of heart disease and stroke) were prevented by interventions that promote healthy lifestyles and environments in youth and throughout adulthood, such efforts would greatly reduce the risk of the current school-aged generation for developing CVD. Testing this hypothesis and others related to CVH promotion and CVD prevention depends on research that is strongly supported, effectively implemented, and adequately sustained. Although current knowledge provides a solid base for policy and practice, more research is needed. Methods for translating existing knowledge into practice must be improved; current and proposed policies and programs that create a demand and opportunity for healthy lifestyles must be evaluated; and new data, especially on social and environmental determinants of CVD, must be collected. These areas correspond closely to the U.S. Department of Health and Human Services priority area of Preventing Disease, Illness, and Injury (Priority X of the Research Themes and Priority Research Areas).[8]

  Theme: A prevention research agenda for heart disease and stroke must be developed and fully implemented to rapidly expand the nation's ability to translate existing knowledge into practice, while continually providing new knowledge to advance public health policy and create more effective programs.

- **Engaging in regional and global partnerships:** Multiplying resources and capitalizing on shared experience (Expert Panel E).

  Perspective: Regional and global partnerships in heart disease and stroke prevention present important opportunities for collaboration, as described in Section 1. Contribution of material and nonmaterial resources developed in the United States can be used to benefit global prevention efforts. Communicating closely with regional and global partners regarding their experiences with policies and programs in diverse settings will be beneficial to all and will return high dividends on investment. Contributions of research in other countries to policy development in the United States are illustrated in Section 1. The threat that CVD poses to human life is important nationally and globally, especially in poorer countries. The widespread occurrence of CVD in countries undergoing social and economic transitions, the unaddressed needs related to CVD prevention, and the need for expanded use of early intervention approaches that are largely unfamiliar all underscore the value of global cooperation.

Theme: As action to prevent heart disease and stroke gains momentum globally, the United States must engage with regional and global partners to support their efforts and to gain from the resulting worldwide growth of knowledge and practical experience.

- **Linking the components:** Integrating the parts and forging a plan (All Expert Panels and the Working Group).

Taking action will be limited initially by the capacity of public health agencies and partners to undertake the work on the scale required. *Strengthening capacity* will enable them to increase the range and intensity of action. *Evaluating impact* will contribute to development of more effective policies and programs, improved identification of best practices, and more rapid communication of new information to the public and policy makers. This activity will increase support for the first two components. *Advancing knowledge* through prevention research will accelerate policy development by supporting critical investigations on policy-related issues and by contributing to better ways to disseminate effective programs widely. Prevention research will become more common as research capacity is strengthened, data systems for surveillance and evaluation are improved, and policy makers increasingly recognize the value of such research. *Regional and global partnerships* will contribute to progress in each of the other four components through the shared experience of global partners who are addressing similar issues.

Theme: Implementation of the plan must assure integration of all five components in a coordinated approach that recognizes and strengthens the potential linkages among them. Such integration and coordination are critical to effective implementation of the plan.

References

1. American Heart Association. *2003 Heart and Stroke Statistics—2003 Update.* Dallas, TX: American Heart Association; 2003.
2. Murray CJL, Lopez A. Alternative Projections of Mortality and Disability by Cause 1990–2020: Global Burden of Disease Study. *Lancet* 1997;349:1498–1504.
3. Association of State and Territorial Directors of Health Promotion and Public Health Education (ASTDHPPHE), and Centers for Disease Control and Prevention (CDC). *Policy and Environmental Change: New Directions for Public Health.* Final Report. Atlanta, GA: ASTDHPPHE and CDC; August 2001.
4. US Department of Health and Human Services. *Healthy People 2010: Understanding and Improving Health and Objectives for Improving Health.* 2nd ed. Vol 1. Washington, DC: US Government Printing Office; November 2000.
5. Committee for the Study of the Future of Public Health, Division of Health Care Services, Institute of Medicine. *The Future of Public Health.* Washington, DC: National Academy Press; 1988.

6. Committee on Educating Public Health Professionals for the 21st Century, Board on Health Promotion and Disease Prevention, Institute of Medicine of the National Academies. Gebbie K, Rosenstock L, Hernandez LM, editors. *Who Will Keep the Public Healthy? Educating Public Health Professionals for the 21st Century*. Washington, DC: The National Academies Press; 2002.

7. Committee on Assuring the Health of the Public in the 21st Century, Board on Health Promotion and Disease Prevention, Institute of Medicine of the National Academies Boufford JI, Cassel CK, co-chairs. *The Future of the Public's Health in the 21st Century*. Washington, DC: The National Academies Press; 2002.

8. Research Coordination Council. *Research Themes and Priority Research Areas*. Washington, DC: US Department of Health and Human Services; 2002 (in press).

SECTION 3.
RECOMMENDATIONS: A CALL TO ACTION

Summary

The *Action Plan* outlines recommendations developed by five Expert Panels that were convened by CDC to address the plan's five essential components. These recommendations were reviewed by a Working Group, which determined that two of the recommendations were paramount and should be elevated above the others as fundamental requirements for implementing this plan (see Appendix D for details of this process). The two fundamental requirements are followed by 22 recommendations, which are presented according to the Expert Panel that produced them.

The Working Group also reviewed the premises that each panel used to guide its recommendations and determined that three of these were relevant to all five components. These were deemed overarching premises and precede the recommendations in this section. All of the other premises outlined by the panels are presented in Appendix D.

Most of the recommendations are directed to the public health community as a whole, especially public health agencies and their partners, which are called to action by this plan. The hope is that all interested agencies, organizations, and individuals will consider these recommendations and the related action steps outlined in Section 4 and will contribute their participation and support.

Overarching Premises

- All recommendations in the plan should contribute to increasing quality and years of healthy life and eliminating health disparities, as well as preventing heart disease and stroke.
- Recommendations should lead to specific actions and measurable outcomes that, when accomplished, will advance the plan. If successful outcomes are effectively communicated, the action steps that led to this success are likely to be replicated throughout the public health system and society at large.
- Because the impact of public health practice is ultimately local (even when the point of action is national or global), the elements required to make a program effective locally should be identified. This process should involve governmental agencies, schools, work sites, communities, families, and other local entities.

Fundamental Requirements

The Working Group determined that two of the Expert Panels' recommendations were paramount and should be elevated above the others as fundamental requirements. These requirements address the crosscutting aspects of effective communication, as well as strategic leadership, partnerships, and organization.

Effective Communication

- **The urgency and promise of preventing heart disease and stroke and their precursors (i.e., atherosclerosis, high blood pressure, and their risk factors and determinants) must be communicated effectively by the public health community through a new long-term strategy of public information and education. This new strategy must engage national, state, and local policy makers and other stakeholders.**

Together, these partners must help the public understand three basic messages. First, heart disease and stroke and related conditions pose a serious threat to the health and well-being of all Americans, especially (but not only) during the middle and older adult years. Second, prevention is possible by reversing community-acquired behaviors, risks, and health disparities. Third, the consequence of failing to intensify preventive efforts is steep escalation in the burden and cost of these diseases in the next two decades and beyond. Success requires a communications infrastructure that includes federal, state, and local public health agencies, tribal organizations, and other government agencies working in partnership with the media and other related sectors.

Communication and education are fundamental to achieving policy and environmental changes, which are strongly recommended in this plan. In addition, policy makers must receive the information necessary to appreciate the urgency of the cardiovascular disease (CVD) epidemic and the opportunity that exists to arrest and reverse it. Leaders in prevention have argued for more than a decade that a broad societal commitment is needed for effective public health efforts to prevent heart disease and stroke. This commitment will depend on critical stakeholders devising and adopting a long-range strategy to convey clear, consistent, and contemporary messages to the public and policy makers.

Strategic Leadership, Partnerships, and Organization

- **The nation's public health agencies and their partners must provide the necessary leadership for a comprehensive public health strategy to prevent heart disease and stroke.**

Appropriate organizational arrangements and sufficient support are needed to achieve effective collaborations among all major partners and to implement the plan. Public health agencies must develop the expertise to create and maintain strong partnerships to advance the agenda for preventing heart disease and stroke at local, state, and national levels. Both traditional and nontraditional partners, including many beyond the health sector, are needed to fully implement the plan.

Strong and committed public health leadership is required to undertake and sustain major new efforts sufficient to arrest and reverse the nation's CVD epidemic. An agency with an appropriate mission, a tradition of relationships with official health agencies and national organizations of public health professionals, and extensive experience in developing and implementing population-wide and community-based health strategies could provide the necessary leadership.

Developing and maintaining effective partnerships requires that public health agencies acquire nontraditional skills and competencies such as knowledge of other relevant organizations and agencies and expertise in communication, collaboration, and negotiation. These skills are presently limited in many if not most public health agencies. When these limitations are overcome, other agencies and organizations in the health sector and in fields that indirectly affect health (e.g., education, agriculture, transportation, community planning) can become engaged in cardiovascular health (CVH) issues and activities.

Recommendations for the Five Essential Components of the Plan

To help the public health community implement the *Action Plan*, specific recommendations were developed by five Expert Panels. These panels addressed the five essential components of the plan—taking action, strengthening capacity, evaluating impact, advancing policy, and engaging in regional and global partnerships. Their work was synthesized by a Working Group into 22 recommendations, which are presented here according to the Expert Panel that produced them.

Taking Action: Putting Present Knowledge to Work

1. **Initiate policy development in CVH promotion and CVD prevention at national, state, and local levels to assure effective public health action against heart disease and stroke. In addition, evaluate policies in non-health sectors (e.g., education, agriculture, transportation, community planning) for their potential impact on health, especially with respect to CVD.**

    As described in Section 1, interventions that address policy and environmental change can have population-wide impact. Such changes represent the coming era of chronic disease prevention and health promotion.[1] The greatest potential for sustained, population-wide health behavior change lies in policy decisions in communities and organizations that support heart-healthy behaviors and in interventions that favor CVH promotion and CVD prevention.

2. **Act now to implement the most promising public health programs and practices for achieving the four goals for preventing heart disease and stroke, as distinguished by the**

Healthy People 2010 Heart and Stroke Partnership based on the different intervention approaches that apply. These goals are prevention of risk factors, detection and treatment of risk factors, early identification and treatment of heart attacks and strokes, and prevention of recurrent cardiovascular events. Public health agencies and their partners must provide continuous leadership to identify and recommend new and effective interventions that are based on advances in program evaluation and prevention research and a growing inventory of "best practices."

To rigorously evaluate policies and programs, new evaluation concepts and methods must continuously be developed. Because input to this development may arise from many sources (e.g., other agencies and organizations, academia, participating communities), establishing leadership responsibility for this function will be advantageous. Taking action based on current knowledge presupposes a well-founded inventory of programs and practices and assessment of their potential effectiveness. Such an inventory is required in relation to the four Healthy People 2010 Heart and Stroke Partnership goals (which are based on the one *Healthy People 2010* goal for preventing heart disease and stroke[2]). Selected programs and practices must also be implemented on a sufficient scale to permit meaningful evaluation of their impact.

3. **Address all opportunities for prevention to achieve the full potential of preventive strategies. Such opportunities include major settings (schools, work sites, health care settings, communities, and families), all age groups (from conception through the life span), and whole populations, particularly priority populations (based on race/ethnicity, sex, disability, economic condition, or place of residence).**

    Only a comprehensive approach can most effectively control the progressive development of risk factors and disease outcomes. In this approach, multiple programs must often be coordinated if all major risk factors are to be addressed in all settings for all population groups. CVH leadership includes assuring that all risk factors are adequately addressed through the available resources and stakeholder groups and that requisite preventive and clinical programs and services of acceptable quality are accessible and used by those who need them.

4. **Emphasize promotion of desirable social and environmental conditions and favorable behavioral patterns in order to prevent the major CVD risk factors and assure the fullest attainable accessibility and use of quality health services for people with risk factors or who develop subclinical or overt CVD. These actions are integral to a comprehensive public health strategy for CVH promotion and CVD prevention.**

Only a comprehensive strategy can effectively address the *Healthy People 2010* goal for preventing heart disease and stroke (see Recommendation 2). Such a strategy for CVH promotion must emphasize the earliest aspects of CVD risk development that jeopardize the health of the entire population (e.g., influences on behavior related to diet; physical activity; and tobacco, alcohol, and drug use) (see Section 2). This is the most neglected area of intervention, and it provides the greatest opportunities both to promote CVH and prevent the later consequences (e.g., risk factors, clinical events). Public health officials and their partners in the health care delivery system and other areas also must assure to the fullest extent possible that clinical guidelines and treatment recommendations for addressing risk factors when they are present (i.e., primary prevention) and CVD events and conditions once they have occurred (i.e., secondary prevention) are implemented effectively across all population groups.

Strengthening Capacity: Transforming the Organization and Structure of Public Health Agencies and Partnerships

5. **Maintain or establish definable entities with responsibility and accountability for CVH programs within federal, state, and local public health agencies, including laboratory components.**

   As a preventable disease that profoundly affects mortality, disability, and health care costs in the United States, CVD warrants visibility and attention as a major public health problem. The large and growing level of disparity among certain racial and ethnic populations adds urgency to this need. Establishing the visibility of CVH in all public health agencies will contribute to the needed recognition of this area of responsibility.

6. **Create a training system to develop and maintain appropriately trained public health workforces at national, state, and local levels. These workforces should have all necessary competencies to bring about policy change and implement programs to improve CVH promotion and decrease the CVD burden, including laboratory requirements.**

   The necessary competencies go beyond traditional public health knowledge to encompass practical skills such as developing and maintaining partnerships and coalitions, defining and identifying the burden and status of chronic diseases, and knowing how to incorporate sound business practices. Few academic training opportunities to learn these essential skills exist in currently available curricula, including master of public health programs. New workers require on-the-job training or other informal means to acquire these skills. Several training options are proposed in Section 4 to meet the needs of local, state, and national public health workers.

7. **Develop and disseminate model performance standards and core competencies in CVD prevention and CVH promotion for national, state, and local public health agencies, including their laboratories.**

   Rather than mandating specific personnel and other resources for CVD prevention programs, setting performance standards and competencies that public health agencies can meet through flexibility with their own personnel and resources may be more successful.

8. **Provide ongoing access to technical assistance and consultation to state and local health agencies and partners for CVD prevention.**

   Although health agencies and organizations can develop personnel capacities through episodic training, continuous availability of technical support through consultation and information sharing can enhance the effectiveness of staff with sufficient previous training. Resources are needed to assure the availability of such support.

Evaluating Impact: Monitoring the Burden, Measuring Progress, and Communicating Urgency

9. **Expand and standardize population-wide evaluation and surveillance data sources and activities to assure adequate assessment of CVD indicators and change in the nation's CVD burden. Examples include mortality, incidence, prevalence, disability, selected biomarkers, risk factors and risk behaviors, economic burden, community and environmental characteristics, current policies and programs, and sociodemographic factors (e.g., age, race/ethnicity, sex, and ZIP code).**

   Existing data sources do not adequately support current population-wide surveillance and evaluation priorities. Strengthening and enhancing these data sources will contribute better information for monitoring and improving CVH in the United States.

10. **Establish a network of data systems for evaluation of policy and program interventions that can track the progress of evolving best practices and signal the need for changes in policies and programs over time. This network would support the full development, collection, and analysis of the data needed to examine program effectiveness.**

    The scientific basis for public health policy and programs in heart disease and stroke prevention must be continually strengthened. A prerequisite for achieving this recommendation is to build data systems that can evaluate health burdens, health practice experiences, and the possible opportunities for new policy and program development.

11. **Develop the public health infrastructure, build personnel competencies, and enhance communication systems so that federal, state, and local public health agencies can communicate surveillance and evaluation results in a timely and effective manner.**

Communicating health information is essential to assuring the timely application of proven interventions for the greatest public health benefit. Strengthening the capacity of public health systems to collect and use information will stimulate policy development and lead to more effective programs and a greater ability to measure their impact.

Advancing Policy: Defining the Issues and Finding the Needed Solutions

12. **Conduct and facilitate research by means of collaboration among interested parties to identify new policy, environmental, and sociocultural priorities for CVH promotion. Once the priorities are identified, determine the best methods for translating, disseminating, and sustaining them. Fund research to identify barriers and effective interventions in order to translate science into practice and thereby improve access to and use of quality health care and improve outcomes for patients with or at risk for CVD. Conduct economics research, including cost-effectiveness studies and comprehensive economic models that assess the return on investment for CVH promotion as well as primary and secondary CVD prevention.**

The importance of policy, environmental, and sociocultural determinants of risk factors and CVD has only been recognized recently and requires intensified investigation. Innovative approaches are needed to advance CVH promotion policy. For example, research is needed to assess community-wide interventions aimed at maintaining and restoring low blood cholesterol levels and low blood pressure, which help prevent atherosclerosis and high blood pressure. To quickly and effectively translate science into practice and improve health outcomes, researchers must identify barriers and implement interventions that prove successful. As the U.S. population ages over the coming decades, the economic aspects of CVD health care (e.g., managing risk factors, events, disabilities, and long-term dependency) will become an even greater problem. Prevention effectiveness research must provide current and projected estimates of the cost to prevent and treat each CVD risk factor and outcome, singly and in integrated multifactor approaches, and determine the cost-effectiveness of current interventions.

13. **Design, plan, implement, and evaluate a comprehensive intervention for children and youth in school, family, and community settings. This intervention must address dietary imbalances, physical inactivity, tobacco use, and other**

determinants in order to prevent development of risk factors and progression of atherosclerosis and high blood pressure.

The need to focus on prevention early in life is compelling. First, very early experience (even in utero or during early postnatal life)[3] may contribute to risk for adult CVD and determine vulnerability to later effects from factors such as weight gain or low income. Second, many health behaviors are established in childhood and youth, when they are more susceptible to change. Third, biological CVD risk factors such as blood cholesterol level and blood pressure and behavioral risk factors such as tobacco use track from childhood into adult life, and family history of CVD predicts CVD risk factors in children and adolescents. Fourth, preclinical CVD in the form of atherosclerosis is already present in youth, and its extent and severity are increased by the presence of these risk factors. Fifth, emerging evidence on biomarkers of risk may point to specific groups especially likely to benefit from intervention. The evidence outlined here indicates that critical, early periods exist when CVD risk can be detected and treated, and research is needed to define these periods more precisely and to demonstrate the impact of population-wide interventions.

14. **Conduct and facilitate research on improvements in surveillance methods and data collection and management methods for policy development, environmental change, performance monitoring, identification of key indicators, and capacity development. Address population subgroups in various settings (schools, work sites, health care, communities) at local, state, and national levels. Additionally, assess the impact of new technologies and regulations on surveillance systems and the potential benefit of alternative methods.**

    Existing surveillance systems do not collect sufficient data in many of these areas. Thus, the ability to make evidence-based improvements in policy and capacity development is limited. Declining survey response rates and increased cell phone use, caller identification technologies, and privacy protections impede collection of data representative of many target populations. Because future innovations could produce communication methods more useful for data collection, methodological research must continue to adapt.

15. **Conduct and support research to determine the most effective marketing messages and educational campaigns to create demand for heart-healthy options, change behavior, and prevent heart disease and stroke for specific target groups and settings. Create and evaluate economically viable CVD prevention ventures (e.g., in food production, manufacturing, marketing).**

    The need for more effective communication about the potential for effective CVH promotion and CVD prevention is widely acknowledged. Research on this topic can contribute substantially to the impact of marketing and public education about heart disease and stroke and increase the return on investment. Strengthening the market for heart-healthy commercial ventures is essential. For example, change in the nation's dietary patterns may require extensive change in food production, processing, marketing, and consumption. Research collaborations that bring interested parties together should achieve a major—if gradual—transition in which public interest and demand for healthy options continue to provide a sustainable economic market for the food industry.

16. **Initiate and strengthen training grants and other approaches, such as training workshops and supervised research opportunities, to build the competencies needed to implement the CVD prevention research agenda.**

Current training programs in prevention research are too few and too small to develop the large cadre of skilled researchers needed to conduct the program effectiveness research and other investigations recommended in this plan. Training grants in other areas have proven that this approach can work.

Engaging in Regional and Global Partnerships: Multiplying Resources and Capitalizing on Shared Experience

17. **Engage with regional and global partners to mobilize resources in CVH promotion and CVD prevention, develop and implement global CVH policies, and establish or strengthen liaison with the partners identified in these recommendations.**

Global partnerships should be strengthened to develop CVH policy and programs that will advance both U.S. and global agendas for enhancing CVH. These efforts can build on existing partnerships, thereby increasing the net investment of effort and resources, and draw on the strengths of the public health community.

18. **Address inequalities in CVH among developed and developing countries, rich and poor people within countries, and men and women of all ages. Work with national and global partners to assess the impact of globalization and trade policies on global CVH.**

Inequalities strongly influence CVH nationally and globally, and eliminating them is a cardinal goal of public health interventions aimed at promoting CVH. Globalization affects many aspects of health among people in the United States and worldwide. Current information on how globalization, including trade policies and practices, affects CVH is inadequate. Better information is needed to determine how the positive forces of globalization can be harnessed to benefit CVH nationally and globally.

19. **Develop a strategy to promote use of the media to support CVH globally.**

    Media channels are powerful health promotion tools that are underused in CVH promotion and CVD prevention. In fact, their messages sometimes serve countervailing interests. Partnership with the global media can help mobilize the use of these capacities to promote CVH.

20. **Strengthen global capacity to develop, implement, and evaluate policy and program interventions to prevent and control heart disease and stroke. Involve all relevant parties—governmental and nongovernmental, public and private, and traditional and nontraditional partners—in a systematic and strategic approach.**

    Improvements in a country's ability to develop or expand its activities in policy and program interventions can best be made if the organizations with experience in this area contribute their expertise. Thus, public health agencies in the United States and their partners can play a significant role in supporting global efforts to prevent and control heart disease and stroke. In addition, partnerships limited only to organizations and agencies within the health sector will be less effective, especially globally, because effective interventions must be multidimensional. Further, the potential for expanding resources and commitments to preventive policies and programs increases as participation grows.

21. **Strengthen the global focus of public health agencies in the United States and their partners on CVH and increase their participation in partnerships intended to a) develop and implement standards for adequate monitoring of health, social, and economic indicators and b) develop the ability to effectively disseminate and translate information into policy and action.**

    A set of standard elements that could or should be collected in a monitoring system is needed. Through technical assistance, public health agencies in the United States and their partners could contribute to this development.

22. **Promote and support research on implementing and evaluating CVH policy interventions in diverse settings where different social and economic development and health transition experiences offer contrasting conditions for testing new intervention approaches.**

    Current research on policy interventions and their impact on CVH promotion and CVD prevention, nationally and globally, is insufficient to provide adequate assurance of their effectiveness. Policy research tools should be developed, and emerging policy interventions that could be useful to the United States and its global partners should be identified and evaluated continually.

References

1. Association of State and Territorial Directors of Health Promotion and Public Health Education (ASTDHPPHE), and Centers for Disease Control and Prevention (CDC). *Policy and Environmental Change: New Directions for Public Health. Final Report*. Atlanta, GA: ASTDHPPHE and CDC; August 2001.
2. US Department of Health and Human Services. *Healthy People 2010: Understanding and Improving Health and Objectives for Improving Health*. 2nd ed. Vol 1. Washington, DC: US Government Printing Office; November 2000.
3. Barker DJP, editor. Fetal and Infant Origins of Adult Disease. London: *British Medical Journal*; 1992.

SECTION 4. IMPLEMENTATION: MOBILIZING FOR ACTION

Summary

Section 3 presented two fundamental requirements and 22 specific recommendations for which action can significantly accelerate progress in preventing heart disease and stroke over the next two decades. To have this impact, each recommendation must be linked with concrete action steps for practical implementation. Such action steps were initially proposed by the Expert Panels, and then reviewed by CDC, a Working Group, and a National Forum convened to help develop this *Action Plan*.

This section presents specific action steps as they correspond to the fundamental requirements and recommendations in Section 3. To indicate their potential impact, the steps are followed by brief descriptions of the outcomes expected from their implementation.

Public health agencies must play leading roles in implementing many or most of the proposed action steps. All steps are addressed implicitly, if not explicitly, to these agencies. All will require broad participation by partner organizations and agencies—public and private—as well as the public health community as a whole. All action steps are directed to all interested and potentially contributing parties. Such partners' commitments are not assumed at this stage of development. Interested organizations and agencies can make these decisions after they have reviewed the plan and identified the areas where they can make the greatest contributions.

This section concludes with a discussion of the immediate need for action, including the initial steps required and the issues that must be addressed, as well as the need for ongoing review, periodic evaluation, and adaptation to future conditions.

Fundamental Action Steps

The two fundamental requirements of this plan and their corresponding action steps address the crosscutting aspects of effective communication, as well as strategic leadership, partnerships, and organization.

Effective Communication

- Assess requirements for effective messages. Set the agenda for a long-term, national public information strategy that conveys the importance and feasibility of prevention. Craft clear and compelling messages that capture public attention, help people understand cardiovascular health (CVH) and its risks, and support healthy behavioral changes. Include a social marketing strategy to identify audiences, develop effective national messages, and determine media avenues (e.g., peer-reviewed journals, CDC's *Morbidity and Mortality Weekly Report*, community report cards). Communicate consistent CVH information and messages to the public, health professionals, and policy makers.

- Communicate effectively at national and state levels to gain consensus on messages and create public demand for heart-healthy options to prevent heart disease and stroke. Work with partners whose roles include education of key stakeholders. Engage local, state, and national policy makers, including new stakeholders.
- Collect information and monitor research systematically from national, state, and local levels to facilitate sharing of knowledge and experience in developing educational campaigns as part of this continuing strategy.

Expected Outcomes
- Communication needs and opportunities are assessed and used to guide initial development of the long-term public information strategy anticipated by the plan.
- Multiple audiences are identified and reached with consistent CVH information and messages. Exposures are targeted and repetitive, reach and maintain critical intensity, neutralize negative messages from special interests, and include expression in popular humor as a measure of public awareness and interest. An effective and sustained communication program exists and is developing appropriate public messages about CVH.
- Public health agencies are promoting continuing development of appropriate educational materials.

Strategic Leadership, Partnerships, and Organization

- Broaden, strengthen, and sustain public health partnerships as an essential force for implementing and institutionalizing the plan. Include public health agencies at all levels (national, state, and local) and a range of other federal, state, and local agencies (e.g., education, agriculture, transportation, housing, environment, tribal organizations); private organizations (e.g., faith-based organizations, business, labor, media, foundations); and academia (e.g., schools of public health, departments of preventive and community medicine, family practice, pediatrics, internal medicine, geriatrics).
- Convene public health agencies at all levels to help develop implementation plans at state and local levels.
- Continue to encourage state health departments to foster internal partnerships and collaborations with complementary CVH-related programs. Allow flexible use of funding to facilitate these important links.
- Explore and enhance the relationships public health agencies have with existing CVH policy coalitions and consider the need for new ones to support the goals of the plan.

Expected Outcomes
- Partnerships supporting the plan are strengthened or established, forming an inclusive array of interests representing all relevant sectors of society.
- State and local public health officials, federal health care systems, and tribal organizations are convened to help implement the plan.
- Support for CVH partnership activities is strengthened, and technical assistance in partnership development and management is available to state and local public health agencies and other interested constituencies. Agencies have expanded the number and diversity of internal and external CVH collaborations. Available funds are used effectively to support coordination among programs.
- Existing CVH policy coalitions are strengthened.

Action Steps for the Five Essential Components

The 22 recommendations presented in Section 3 require specific action steps to guide implementation of the plan. This section outlines action steps proposed by the Expert Panels and synthesized by the Working Group. They are presented in the same order as the plan's five essential components, which are taking action, strengthening capacity, evaluating impact, advancing policy, and engaging in regional and global partnerships. Each group of action steps is followed by expected outcomes that indicate their potential impact.

Taking Action: Putting Present Knowledge to Work

1. **Initiate policy development.**
   - Establish active collaboration among public health agencies, clinical preventive service providers, and other partners at all levels (e.g., purchasers of health care insurance, insurers, providers of care, health counselors, patient groups) to implement effective policies and programs that address CVH promotion and primary and secondary prevention of cardiovascular disease (CVD).
   - Develop and regularly update simulation models to address the expected health and economic benefits to society from investing in heart disease and stroke prevention.
   - Conduct health impact assessments of national policies and provide a framework to states to conduct these assessments at the state level.

   Expected Outcomes
   - Through technical assistance, consultation, and cooperative arrangements, partners who deliver CVH promotion and CVD prevention programs and services at all levels are receiving active support and incentives. These partners are developing and implementing more effective policies that address the full spectrum of intervention approaches

represented in the action framework in Section 2 and reflect current knowledge of the efficacy and safety of therapeutic interventions.

- Comprehensive economic modeling of the CVD burden and the potential impact of preventive policies and programs is ongoing and supports policy development and implementation.

- National, state, and local policies are regularly identified and subject to health impact assessments with specific attention to their potential effects on CVH and other chronic diseases of public health concern.

2. **Implement best practices.**
   - Review, revise if appropriate, and rigorously apply criteria for identifying model programs. In the meantime, implement current programs and evaluate them against these criteria.
   - Identify and disseminate information about model programs that include all elements of best practices for a population-based approach to CVH. Test the synergistic effects of composite programs.
   - Generate and test new intervention models by funding new demonstration projects. Share materials and experiences in order to continually develop, implement, and evaluate best practices.

   Expected Outcomes
   - Criteria appropriate for identifying best practices in CVH promotion and CVD prevention are established and are being used. Programs considered the most promising are implemented as expeditiously as possible, with adequate provision for rigorously evaluating these programs in accordance with accepted criteria.
   - These criteria are applied continually to identify model CVH/CVD programs, especially those in which multiple components are coordinated and integrated for maximum impact. These model programs are being disseminated.
   - Innovative demonstration programs are being funded and rigorously evaluated. The resulting experiences are communicated rapidly and effectively to facilitate program replication and dissemination.

3. **Address prevention in all settings, life stages, and priority populations.**
   - Develop, implement, and evaluate programs to address opportunities for CVH promotion and CVD prevention in the full array of multiple settings (e.g., schools, work sites, health care settings, other community sites), during all life stages (gestation; infancy and childhood; adolescence; and early, middle, and late adulthood), and among all priority populations (as defined by excessive health burdens or needs).

Expected Outcomes
- A matrix of settings, life stages, and at-risk populations is developed and disseminated as a tool for identifying policy and program needs and opportunities. Model policies and programs to address the demonstrated needs and opportunities are identified (or developed) and evaluated. These model policies and programs are disseminated for implementation at national, state, and local levels.

4. **Accept the full scope of public health responsibility.**
   - Accept accountability of public health agencies, their partners, and society as a whole for addressing the full spectrum of opportunities to prevent heart disease and stroke as part of a comprehensive public health strategy.
   - Collaborate with partners in related fields (e.g., nutrition, physical activity, tobacco control, substance abuse), including those working to detect and treat risk factors (e.g., hyperlipidemia, high blood pressure, smoking, diabetes, obesity). Support programmatic activities in schools, work sites, health care settings, and community sites and for priority populations.
   - Establish or strengthen collaborations with the Centers for Medicare & Medicaid Services, the National Committee for Quality Assurance, and other partners positioned to improve access to and use of high-quality care for patients with or at risk for CVD.

Expected Outcomes
- CVH programs are recognized as having responsibility and accountability for a comprehensive public health strategy that addresses the full array of approaches to CVH promotion and CVD prevention, to help achieve the four Healthy People 2010 Heart and Stroke Partnership goals for preventing heart disease and stroke.
- The needed partnerships and collaborations are in place at national, state, and local levels to support these activities.
- Partnerships are strengthened or established with the full array of organizations and agencies committed to effectively delivering high-quality health services (including preventive services) as part of a comprehensive public health strategy.

Strengthening Capacity: Transforming the Organization and Structure of Public Health Agencies and Partnerships

5. **Establish CVH entities within public health agencies.**
   - Transform public health agencies at all levels so they can effectively prevent heart disease and stroke.
   - Establish or strengthen identifiable CVH units in public health agencies at all levels. These units should be able to effectively reach all communities and have all necessary capacities for preventing heart disease and stroke, including new competencies

in policy and environmental change, population-wide health promotion and behavioral change for risk factor prevention, and early detection and control of risk factors.

Expected Outcomes
- Public health agencies throughout the nation are undergoing the changes needed to expand their roles and meet the new challenges of preventing heart disease and stroke and other chronic conditions of public health concern.
- Every state and territorial health agency has an identifiable unit or locus of responsibility for CVH policy and programs. These agencies are able to provide support and assistance in CVH activities to all local health agencies within their jurisdictions. Through increased and creative collaborations, public health agencies and their partners are strengthening their efforts to promote CVH and prevent risk factors and first CVD events.

6. **Reinvent innovative training resources and opportunities.**
    - Develop training resources, including technical assistance and materials, to enable states to train staff in state and local health departments and in partner organizations and agencies, assuring that they have core competencies and meet performance standards in CVH. These include changes in organizational structure, skills in incorporating best practices, and assurance of partnership effectiveness.
    - Establish training in the following set of skills, which are essential to an effective public health workforce:
        - Developing and maintaining partnerships and coalitions.
        - Promoting community mobilization for effective action.
        - Using health communications effectively.
        - Defining and identifying the burden and status of chronic diseases.
        - Preventing and managing risk factors.
        - Formulating and executing policy and environmental approaches to intervention.
        - Organizing effective prevention programs.
        - Leading diverse community organizations.
        - Conducting culturally appropriate interventions targeted to priority populations.
        - Using sound business practices and strategic planning to improve public health.
    - Consider a variety of options for training personnel. Possibilities include the following:
        - Schools of public health and other professional schools in health fields.
        - Train-the-trainer programs (e.g., in the use of data for health planning, health promotion, primary and secondary prevention, program planning, and evaluation, including population-based interventions).
        - A certificate program in CVH.
        - CVH training at Prevention Research Centers.

- CVH training programs with standard curricula.
- An expanded year-round program implemented with state and local health agencies.
- Joint school health/public health courses.
- Regional networks for education and training.
- Internet training programs.
- Continuing education, including training in information technology.

- Involve numerous partners, such as directors of state chronic disease programs, voluntary associations, and academic institutions, in the development of training programs. Sample activities include the following:
  - Allow all state and local health agencies access to training and development opportunities, information, and materials regardless of their funding status.
  - Provide state and local health personnel and partners access to professional development opportunities.
  - Tailor training programs to the concerns, interests, and needs of local, state, and national constituents.
  - Provide training in chronic disease prevention to personnel from diverse organizations, including governmental agencies, public health and education, schools of public health, and nongovernmental health organizations.

Expected Outcomes
- A comprehensive CVH training function is developed and coordinated among all interested parties, providing a resource for state and local health agencies.
- Model curricula and educational programs (e.g., Web-based, video training packages) are available, including those needed for developing nontraditional skills. Trainees in target areas are meeting established goals.
- Training programs for CVH public health personnel are identified. State and regional networks for CVH training and education are established to coordinate training needs with available resources.
- Model education and training programs are being developed and disseminated to state and local health agencies and partners.

7. **Develop and disseminate standards.**
   - Develop performance standards and cultural competency guidelines for public health agencies and partners. Include maintenance of laboratory capacity and standardizations. Share these with schools of public health and other educational sources for health professionals and encourage their adoption in curricula.
   - Identify mechanisms (e.g., technical assistance, dedicated funding and staff) that enable local and state health departments to meet standards.

Expected Outcomes

- Performance standards and cultural competency guidelines for CVH programs are established to help public health agencies transcend "business as usual" and undertake new directions in public health practice. Existing mandates are maintained, and efforts are expanded in early intervention (i.e., policy and environmental change; behavioral change; and prevention, detection, and control of risk factors). Laboratory capacity to address emerging issues is enhanced. Public health agencies are communicating with schools of public health and other training programs regarding training and curriculum requirements for public health personnel working in CVH and related program areas.
- Public health agencies are receiving technical assistance in monitoring and improving cultural competency in CVH and related program areas.

8. **Provide technical support.**
   - Develop and maintain a cadre of educated practitioners and technical experts who can support intervention needs in CVH promotion and CVD prevention (i.e., surveillance, trend analysis, behavior change, community development). Draw these practitioners and experts from local, state, and national public health agencies, as well as from voluntary health associations, academia, foundations, and a variety of industries. Assure the means for keeping their skills up-to-date (e.g., through meetings and Web-based curricula).
   - Develop materials and tools to promote CVH at local and state levels.
   - Strengthen the internal communications infrastructure of public health agencies for chronic disease programs as they make other general infrastructure improvements.

   ## *Expected Outcomes*

   - A register of recognized experts willing to provide technical and policy assistance to local, state, and federal health agencies and other CVH partners is established and maintained. Use of the registry is supported and monitored. Training and educational opportunities are provided, and the registered experts use them.
   - State and local health agency needs for CVH promotional materials and an educational "toolbox" are being met.
   - A public health communications infrastructure supportive of CVH (and other chronic disease) activities is in place and is continually adopting newer, more effective communications technology.

Evaluating Impact: Monitoring the Burden, Measuring Progress, and Communicating Urgency

9. **Expand and standardize population-wide data sources and activities.**
    *   Define the characteristics of surveillance and evaluation systems at minimal, desirable, and optimal levels. Establish an inclusive framework and set of indicators on the basis of 1) a review of existing surveillance and evaluation frameworks (e.g., the World Health Organization's STEPwise approach, Canada's recent development of surveillance priorities); 2) the new requirements for monitoring policy and environmental change; behavioral change; biomarkers of CVD risk; and risk factor prevention, detection, and control; and 3) input from national, state, and local stakeholders and partner organizations. Include social and environmental science and policy experts and those who collect, analyze, or use relevant data.
    *   Assess the adequacy of current systems on the basis of these characteristics and the need for dynamic, interactive data access and use. Include the experts and stakeholders described in the previous action step.
    *   Convene public health agencies and partners to determine the mechanisms and costs needed to fill identified information gaps. Improve existing data sets and develop new ones as needed, with attention to timeliness, sustainability, and standardization. Address standardization of data systems across states, approaches to active or passive data collection, ongoing versus episodic data collection requirements, availability of data from health care insurers, and the paramount importance of incidence data for monitoring progress in preventing heart disease and stroke. Devise common data formats, data management policies and practices, and methods for controlling interconnected data systems.
    *   Use data to plan health programs and to communicate consistent messages about the urgency of preventing heart disease and stroke. Enhance the incorporation of current CVH data into broader social indicator reports, using model programs and tested tools, formats, and templates for communicating and disseminating this information.

    ### *Expected Outcomes*
    *   A framework is reviewed and established for assessing data requirements for monitoring and evaluating the comprehensive public health strategy. It includes a mechanism for periodic updates and reassessments.
    *   An initial inventory of health indicators (including applicable leading health indicators from *Healthy People 2010*) and relevant surveillance and evaluation data sources is completed and disseminated to appropriate agencies and organizations for review and comment.

- A group has convened and formulated a detailed implementation plan for developing the monitoring and evaluation data systems needed to support the *Action Plan.*
- As the available data are used to communicate CVH messages, their strengths and limitations and the current systems for managing and coordinating these data are continuously monitored. System development is advanced and adapted to changing needs.

10. **Establish data systems for evaluation of policy and program interventions.**
    - Assure that resources are allocated when projects or model programs are first funded by public health agencies and partners (e.g., personnel or financial set-asides) to permit adequate evaluation of outcomes and costs.
    - Develop guidelines for public health agencies and partners for content and format of such evaluations, especially in the new areas of policy and environmental change; behavioral change; and risk factor prevention, detection, and control.

    Expected Outcomes
    - Evaluation is an expected component of every public health program aimed at preventing heart disease and stroke. No program proceeds without commitment to support this component.
    - Tools are widely available to support evaluations and the timely communication of their findings. This allows the most effective interventions to be replicated quickly. Mechanisms for disseminating and reviewing evaluation results are strengthened to assure that the knowledge and experience gained are applied in future policies and programs.

11. **Develop professional staff capacity for monitoring and evaluation.**
    - Strengthen the surveillance and program evaluation functions of public health agencies through enhanced staffing and resources, especially for monitoring policy and environmental change; behavioral change; and risk factor prevention, detection, and control.
    - Provide guidance to state and local health agencies and partners regarding capacity requirements for surveillance and evaluation activities.
    - Establish resources to support program evaluation through training, consultation, technical assistance, and partnerships to develop logic models, methodology, data collection, and reporting.

    Expected Outcomes
    - Professional staff development for monitoring and evaluation, especially in the new areas required by the plan, is

a priority for all public health agencies, which have expanded their capacity for advancing methods and practices in CVH program evaluation.

- State and local public health agencies are receiving help in determining what capacities they need to evaluate their programs.
- A plan for meeting these requirements is developed and implemented.

Advancing Policy: Defining the Issues and Finding the Needed Solutions

12. Conduct and facilitate policy and environmental research.

- Focus on preventing atherosclerosis and high blood pressure. Develop and support a collaborative, detailed, and interdisciplinary research agenda and a new framework for policy, environmental, and behavioral research to determine which interventions (separately or in combination) will best affect atherosclerosis and high blood pressure and their contribution to the burden of heart disease and stroke. Support both targeted and investigator-initiated research.
- Support research to determine the best ways to implement and disseminate the most effective policy, environmental, or behavioral change interventions to prevent heart disease and stroke. Identify social and cultural factors that promote or inhibit the sustainability of interventions, especially among populations affected by disparities in CVD risk (based on race/ethnicity, income, or place of residence).
- Conduct research to answer questions such as the following: What are the social and structural factors in various settings and sectors that affect CVH status more than individual characteristics? What are specific antecedent factors associated with specific components of risk (e.g., food intake, physical activity, adherence to preventive medical care)? What are the social and cultural determinants of food consumption and physical activity among children and families? How do these factors differ by characteristics such as age, income, or race? What is the public health importance of currently available genetic and other biomarkers of risk or disease?
- Develop and support a collaborative research agenda that focuses on health outcomes. Establish effective interventions to overcome barriers and improve access to and use of high-quality medical services for patients with or at risk for heart disease and stroke.
- Support prevention effectiveness research to determine what combinations of effective interventions (e.g., policy, environment, individual) at what doses, in what settings (e.g., family, school, work site, health care, community), at what life stages, and among which priority populations are most effective in preventing, detecting, and controlling CVD risk factors.

- Express strong support for this new research agenda with the help of partners positioned to educate key stakeholders, to help policy makers recognize its value, and to assure its implementation and the continual advancement of resulting policies and programs.

Expected Outcomes
- A research agenda specific to the major focus of preventing atherosclerosis and high blood pressure is developed and implemented.
- A detailed research agenda is developed and supported, in alignment with the Research Themes and Research Priority Areas of the U.S. Department of Health and Human Services, with special emphasis on policy and environmental change related to CVH promotion and CVD prevention.
- A broad array of relevant research questions is developed and prioritized to balance the research agenda.
- The research agenda includes studies to identify potential points of intervention to improve preventive services and access to and use of these services. This agenda supports the four goals for preventing heart disease and stroke as distinguished by the Healthy People 2010 Heart and Stroke Partnership. These goals are prevention of risk factors, detection and treatment of risk factors, early detection and treatment of heart attacks and strokes, and prevention of recurrent cardiovascular events.
- The research agenda includes studies involving the proposed matrix of settings, life stages, and priority populations to determine the most effective interventions within and across populations (including population-wide approaches and those aimed a specific subgroups).
- The research agenda is supported by education to assure that funding is a national priority.

13. Prevent risk factors in youth and beyond.
- Develop and support detailed research agendas that specifically address prevention in youth and early adulthood. Include studies that assess the impact of known interventions in preventing risk factors, atherosclerosis, and high blood pressure.
- Identify subclinical indicators of CVD and potentially useful genetic and other biomarkers that can be applied in population studies and prevention programs. Work with appropriate health service and industry partners.
- Identify other outstanding concerns in preventing risk factors.

Expected Outcomes
- A detailed research agenda is developed and supported to design, implement, and evaluate intervention programs to prevent CVD risk factors, atherosclerosis, and high blood pressure, beginning in childhood.

- This agenda includes research to develop assessment methods for subclinical atherosclerosis and to evaluate new candidate biomarkers in population studies, especially during adolescence and early adulthood.
- The agenda includes research on underlying determinants of CVD risk factors. Examples include how fetal development affects later risk and how nutrition and physical activity affect obesity, blood lipids, and blood pressure.

14. Conduct and facilitate monitoring and evaluation research.

- Support monitoring and evaluation research to determine how best to measure policy and environmental change interventions.
- Incorporate these measures into surveillance systems.
- Respond to technological developments and regulations that restrict access to personal health information to assure the appropriate levels of participation and representation in surveillance activities.

Expected Outcomes

- The research agenda includes studies of methods and data requirements for monitoring and evaluating approaches to policy and environmental change.
- Surveillance methods that incorporate the relevant data elements are developed and implemented.
- Methods that assure adequate participation rates and representative population samples are continuously investigated, addressing technical and policy concerns about access to health information.

15. Conduct and support marketing research.

- Support marketing research on how to inform the public effectively and bring about health behavioral change.
- Support research to demonstrate the economic feasibility of and appropriate business models for private-sector investment in prevention (e.g., in food production, manufacturing, or marketing).

Expected Outcomes

- The research agenda includes studies of what influences the way people respond to population-wide and individual interventions to prevent heart disease and stroke in the community at large, in specific cultural communities, and in specific organizational settings.
- The research agenda includes studies of how consumer products could be changed to support policies and programs to reduce risk for heart disease and stroke and still be viable commercially. This research includes partners in business and industry.

16. Strengthen the prevention research workforce.

- Inventory current prevention research training programs and research opportunities in view of the expanding need for new health research skills.

- Emphasize policy and environmental change, health behavioral change, and risk factor prevention when seeking to identify training needs and develop responsive plans.

Expected Outcomes

- Workforce requirements for establishing and maintaining broad-based CVH prevention research programs are documented. Training programs to meet current and future requirements are identified and evaluated.
- Gaps in training resources are identified, and detailed plans for filling them are developed. Resources are identified and committed to support the needed training in CVH prevention research.

Engaging in Regional and Global Partnerships: Multiplying Resources and Capitalizing on Shared Experience

17. Provide global leadership, partnerships, and organization.

- Develop and effectively support a global mission and vision of the United States for CVH.
- Inventory existing and potential partners for global CVH collaboration, with support from public health agencies and other partners. Include governmental agencies, nongovernmental organizations, and foundations (e.g., especially the World Health Organization, World Heart Federation, and World Bank).
- Evaluate current CVH research and training programs of these potential partners. Evaluate their interest in receiving information and technical support from public health agencies to enhance these programs and in planning joint projects or programs. Include entities with policy roles that might conflict with CVH priorities, but who could become effective partners (e.g., the food and agriculture sector).

Expected Outcomes

- A statement of the U.S. position, role, and interest regarding global CVH needs and opportunities has been published and serves as a point of reference for partnership development in this area.
- Inventories of existing regional and global CVH partnerships, potential nontraditional CVH partnerships, and foundations that support international activities for medical and public health training are established and maintained.
- An inventory of current agendas for integrated CVH research, linked with other chronic conditions of public health importance, is established and maintained. Joint projects with regional and global partners are planned and implemented.

18. Establish and support global policies.

- Establish a partnership for global heart disease and stroke that develops, monitors, and evaluates global CVH strategy.
- Focus on eliminating inequalities in CVH in the United States and globally, and assess the contribution of this country's global strategy in reducing CVH inequalities worldwide.
- Assess the impact of globalization and trade policies (e.g., related to tobacco, food and agriculture, and pharmaceuticals) on national and international trends in CVD and suggest improvements that could favorably affect CVH.

  Expected Outcomes
  - A partnership on global CVH strategy is established. Its implementation plan is guided by a commitment to work toward eliminating inequalities in CVH.
  - A framework to assess progress on equity in national and global CVH programs is being used.
  - Study results are published on the impact of globalization and trade policies (especially those related to tobacco, food, and pharmaceuticals) on CVH, as well as the opportunities to harness these policies to promote CVH nationally and globally.

19. Develop a global communications strategy.

- Establish relationships between transnational media organizations and public health agencies and partners to identify models of collaboration that can help improve media content and coverage on the need for global CVH promotion and CVD prevention.
- Effectively communicate to health professionals throughout the world that they should promote CVH by supporting effective policies and by serving as role models for positive behavioral patterns.

  Expected Outcomes
  - Consensus development meetings are conducted among CVH partners and media representatives. Better CVH messages are communicated through the media.
  - Programs are undertaken to reach health professionals throughout the world with effective messages about their role in preventing heart disease and stroke.

20. Strengthen global capacity.

- Develop tailored programs to 1) assist and support decision makers interested in developing and implementing effective national policies, 2) develop methodology and tools to analyze the health impact of policy interventions, and 3) analyze the social and economic costs of heart disease and stroke and the benefits of preventing them.
- Promote the exchange of information and experiences on policies that promote CVH.

- Collect existing tools for assessing policy and environmental change and program effectiveness, synthesize an integrated assessment tool, apply this tool to identify best practices, and increase information sharing through technology.
- Develop and implement strategies to assure that changes that support the *Action Plan* are institutionalized.

Expected Outcomes

- Development of capacity for heart disease and stroke prevention is recognized as a long-term requirement for transforming public health agencies. The proposed training programs and workshops are available and being used. International conferences are conducted on the economics of heart disease and stroke prevention and the links between economic conditions and CVH.
- Information and experience related to CVH promotion are effectively disseminated and applied (e.g., the *International Action on Cardiovascular Disease: A Platform for Success*, published by the World Heart Federation and the International Heart Health Society).
- Tools for analyzing how policies affect the global dimensions of CVH are developed and disseminated.
- Capacity is developed in a way that assures institutionalization of change.

21. Strengthen global monitoring and evaluation.

- Inventory existing surveys, programs, and agreements relevant to global activities in heart disease and stroke prevention and control.
- Identify existing programs that could be expanded and areas where new collaborations could be created. This activity could be conducted by organizations such as CDC, the World Health Organization (WHO), the World Heart Federation, the Pan American Health Organization, and the InterAmerican Heart Foundation.
- Support monitoring of heart disease and stroke globally by working with existing and new partners (especially WHO) to develop standard data elements. These elements should include 1) mortality, morbidity, and risk factors; 2) nontraditional elements such as clinical factors (e.g., patterns of diagnosis, treatment, use); 3) preventive and health promotion programs; and 4) social, cultural, environmental, and policy factors. Assure effective dissemination of the resulting information and its translation into action.

Expected Outcomes

- A Web-based inventory is available and routinely updated.
- New regional and global collaborative activities are established, and new opportunities are being identified.
- Guidelines for standard data collection and methods for planning and evaluating heart disease and stroke prevention

and control programs are developed and being used. Training programs for technical assistance/collaboration on CVD projects are receiving needed financial support.

22. Promote and support global research.
- Collaborate in developing a research agenda on CVH policy. Identify appropriate international partners to design research and mobilize resources.

Expected Outcomes
- Public health agencies are actively designing and conducting policy research to identify best practices for preventing heart disease and stroke in diverse socioeconomic settings, both nationally and globally.

Steps Toward Implementation

To make the *Action Plan* a reality, action is needed now. Mobilizing this action requires detailed plans of implementation; methods for measuring short-, mid-, and long-term outcomes and impacts; and a process for oversight and evaluation.

Close collaboration with public health agencies at state, territorial, local, and tribal levels is needed. These collaborations can 1) promote development of specific implementation plans; 2) align partnerships to broaden and deepen the base of support for the *Action Plan* and strengthen overall capacity; 3) provide comprehensive, timely, and accurate data to guide policy and decision makers, health professionals, and the public; and 4) provide appropriate interaction among partners in the scientific community to advance prevention effectiveness research to evaluate policies and programs.

Review, Evaluation, and Adaptation to Future Conditions

To assure long-term success, the need to review and evaluate all aspects of the plan and adapt it to future conditions must be anticipated. For example, we must consider the projected demographic shift toward an increasingly older U.S. population and the expected increase in demand for health services by the population as a whole. These recognized factors were considered when the recommendations for this plan were developed. However, other contingencies resulting from unforeseen social and economic forces may require significant adaptations over the next two decades.

For this and other reasons, an explicit evaluation process must be designed and implemented. This evaluation plan must include the following elements: 1) a comprehensive logic model as the basis for evaluation; 2) short-, mid-, and long-term evaluation criteria; 3) key indicators and data systems; 4) procedures for evaluation, as well as for reporting and updating key assumptions and projections; and 5) responsibility and authority for revising the plan. Substantial work remains to be done to develop detailed implementation plans for each of the *Action Plan's* five essential components and to initiate the needed actions. But great progress has been made by bringing the plan to completion at this stage.

The *Action Plan* provides a view of the current reality concerning the nation's burden of heart disease and stroke, a vision of a future in which the epidemic occurrence of these conditions has been controlled, and an understanding of the wide range of intervention approaches that can and must be applied to achieve this vision. The plan also identifies key issues and proposes recommendations and specific action steps in five essential areas. This information is presented in the context of a comprehensive public health strategy to prevent heart disease and stroke in the United States and contribute to similar efforts with global partners. By implementing these recommendations, the nation's public health agencies—strengthened by a broad array of partnerships reflecting society's interest in preventing these diseases—can undergo significant positive transformation in their roles and accomplish major progress in preventing heart disease and stroke. Expanding from traditional roles to embrace new opportunities for health impact, through policy and environmental change and health behavioral change, these agencies can succeed in making sure that the nation is as healthy as possible.

APPENDIX A: GLOSSARY

The following brief definitions or explanations apply to technical or common terms used specifically in the *Action Plan*. For more detailed definitions, standard reference works should be consulted.

acute case management: an intervention approach in which individual cardiovascular disease (CVD) events (e.g., heart attack, heart failure, stroke) are treated as they occur.

age-adjusted death rate: the number of deaths occurring per 100,000 population per year, calculated in accordance with a standard age structure to minimize the effect of age differences when rates are compared between populations or over time.

Alzheimer's disease: the most common cause of dementia, or decline in mental function, characterized by degeneration of nerve cells and loss of brain substance, most common among people older than age 65 years.

assessment: the obligation of every public health agency to monitor the health status and needs of its community regularly and systematically; one of the three core functions of public health.

assurance: the guarantee of governments that agreed-upon, high-priority, personal and community health services will be provided to every member of the community by qualified organizations; one of the three core functions of public health.

atheroma: a concentrated area of mushy material within the wall of an artery, often encrusted or hardened (sclerosed) by deposited calcium, that is the pathological hallmark of atherosclerosis.

atherosclerosis: a pathological condition affecting the medium-sized and larger arteries, especially those that supply the heart (the coronary arteries), the brain (the carotid and cerebral arteries), and the lower extremities (the peripheral arteries), as well as the aorta; underlies the occurrence of heart attacks, many strokes, peripheral arterial disease, and dissection or rupture of the aorta.

behavioral change: an intervention approach that uses public information and education to promote behavioral patterns favorable to health for the population as a whole; also includes interventions (e.g., counseling) at the group or individual level for the same purpose.

behavioral patterns: habits of living (e.g., diet, physical activity, smoking) that influence health.

blood cholesterol: the blood concentration of a family of lipid or "fatty" molecular compounds obtained directly from the diet or produced in the body from fatty dietary components; a necessary factor in development of atherosclerosis; total cholesterol concentration is classified as "high" if it is ≥200 mg/dl. Subtypes of cholesterol differ in their relation to CVD risk, with high-density lipoprotein (HDL) cholesterol considered "good," and low-density (LDL) cholesterol considered "bad."

blood pressure: see *high blood pressure*.

cardiovascular disease prevention: a set of interventions designed to prevent first and recurrent CVD events (e.g., heart attack, heart failure, stroke). For CVD, *primary prevention* refers to detection and control of risk factors, whereas *secondary prevention* includes long-term case management for survivors of CVD events. CVD prevention complements cardiovascular health (CVH) promotion.

cardiovascular disease(s): may refer to any of the disorders that can affect the circulatory system, but often means coronary heart disease (CHD), heart failure, and stroke, taken together.

cardiovascular health: a combination of favorable health habits and conditions that protects against development of cardiovascular diseases.

cardiovascular health promotion: a set of interventions designed to reduce a population's risk for CVD through policy, environmental, and behavioral changes; also supports other approaches that apply to people who have suffered recognized CVD events (e.g., by facilitating public access to emergency care or by fostering social/environmental and behavioral changes that reinforce *secondary CVD prevention*); sometimes identified with *primordial CVD prevention*; complements CVD prevention.

carotid arteries: the four main arteries of the head and neck, which supply blood to the brain and elsewhere in the head.

case fatality rate: the proportion of cases of a disease event ending in death within a defined interval (e.g., 41% of those experiencing a first heart attack die within 28 days of onset of the attack).

cerebral arteries: blood vessels connecting the internal carotid arteries with the brain.

cerebral hemorrhage: rupture of a cerebral blood vessel, characterized by accumulation of blood at the site of the rupture and loss of blood supply beyond the point of rupture, often leading to a sudden focal loss of brain function or stroke.

cholesterol: see *blood cholesterol*.

chronic kidney (renal) disease: long-term impairment of kidney function often leading to high blood pressure or kidney failure; may be treated with medication, kidney transplantation, or dialysis.

circulatory system: the network of arteries, veins, capillaries, and lymphatic vessels throughout the body, including the heart, that pumps blood to the lungs and peripheral tissues.

comprehensive public health strategy: an approach to a major health problem in the population that identifies and employs the full array of potential public health interventions, including health promotion and disease prevention.

congestive heart failure: see *heart failure*.

core functions of public health: the three main areas of responsibility of official public health agencies as defined by the Committee for the Study of the Future of Public Health: assessment, policy development, and assurance.

coronary arteries: the arteries that supply blood to the heart muscle and whose narrowing or occlusion constitutes coronary heart disease and can precipitate a heart attack.

coronary heart disease: heart disease caused by impaired circulation in one or more coronary arteries; often manifests as chest pain (angina pectoris) or heart attack.

CVD prevention: see *cardiovascular disease prevention*.

CVH promotion: see *cardiovascular health promotion*.

diabetes (or diabetes mellitus): a metabolic disorder resulting from insufficient production or utilization of insulin, commonly leading to cardiovascular complications.

diastolic blood pressure: see *high blood pressure*.

dietary imbalance: a pattern of dietary intake that lacks a desirable combination and overall intake of foods and nutrients to promote good health (e.g., excessive intake of saturated fat, salt, total calories).

disparities: see *health disparities*.

economic development: the long-term process of economic growth in developing countries or economically disadvantaged areas of developed countries; can influence the health of residents favorably or unfavorably.

emergency care: treatment for people who have experienced a first or recurrent acute CVD event (e.g., heart attack, heart failure, stroke) designed to increase their probability of survival and to minimize associated damage or disability.

end-of-life care: treatment for late or terminal complications of CVD designed to minimize suffering and preserve the dignity of those treated.

epidemiology: the study of the causes and prevention of disease in populations or communities, making it the main source of evidence for public health decision making.

evidence-based medicine: the use of agreed-upon standards of evidence in making clinical decisions for treating individual patients or categories of patients.

evidence-based public health: the use of agreed-upon standards of evidence in making decisions about public health policies and practices to protect or improve the health of populations.

health disparities: differences in the burden and impact of disease among different populations, defined, for example, by sex, race or ethnicity, education or income, disability, place of residence, or sexual orientation.

Healthy People 2010: a document that presents health-related goals and objectives for the United States to be achieved by the year 2010.

Healthy People 2010 Heart and Stroke Partnership: established to achieve the *Healthy People 2010* goal for preventing heart disease and stroke. The members of the partnership divided this goal into four separate ones: prevention of risk factors, detection and treatment of risk factors, early detection and treatment of heart attacks and strokes, and prevention of recurrent cardiovascular events. This partnership was established by the American Heart Association/American Stroke Association, Centers for Disease Control and Prevention, Centers for Medicare & Medicaid Services, National Institutes of Health, and Office of Public Health and Science, U.S. Department of Health and Human Services.

heart attack: an acute event in which the heart muscle is damaged because of a lack of blood flow from the coronary arteries, typically accompanied by chest pain and other warning signs but sometimes occurring with no recognized symptoms (i.e., "silent heart attack").

heart disease: any affliction that impairs the structure or function of the heart (e.g., athero-sclerotic and hypertensive diseases, congenital heart disease, rheumatic heart disease, and cardiomyopathies).

Heart Disease and Stroke Control Program: a program established by the National Heart Act of 1948 through which the federal government supported state efforts to prevent and control heart disease and stroke; terminated in 1970.

Heart Disease and Stroke Prevention Program: a CDC program initiated in 1998 that supports states in their efforts to prevent heart disease and stroke; for more information see www.cdc.gov/cvh/stateprogram.htm.

heart failure: impairment of the pumping function of the heart as the result of heart disease; heart failure often causes physical disability and increased risk for other CVD events.

high blood pressure: a condition in which the pressure in the arterial circulation is greater than desired; associated with increased risk for heart disease, stroke, chronic kidney disease, and other conditions; blood pressure is considered "high" if systolic pressure (measured at the peak of contraction of the heart) is ≥140 mm Hg or if diastolic pressure (measured at the fullest relaxation of the heart) is ≥90 mm Hg.

high-risk approach: an intervention strategy that targets only people with the highest levels of recognized CVD risk factors for the purpose of reducing their level of risk to that of the most favorable level in the population; distinct from and complementary to the *population-wide approach*.

hypertension: see *high blood pressure*.

hypertensive heart disease: abnormality in the structure and function of the heart caused by long-standing high blood pressure; often manifests as heart failure.

incidence: the number of new cases of disease occurring in a population of given size within a specified time interval (e.g., the average annual incidence of stroke for women in Rochester, Minnesota, during 1985–1989 was approximately 120/100,000 population).

individual approach: see *high-risk approach*.

Inter-Society Commission for Heart Disease Resources: a commission established under U.S. Public Law 89-239 as part of the Regional Medical Programs Service; responsible for producing guidelines defining optimal medical resources and care for the prevention and treatment of cardiovascular diseases in the United States.

life cycle: the course of human development from conception until death, including gestation; infancy; childhood; adolescence; and early, middle, and late adulthood; important for targeting health promotion and disease prevention efforts to the distinct needs of people in each phase.

long-term case management: an intervention approach that targets survivors of CVD events; designed to reduce disability and the risk for recurrent events.

modifiable characteristics: factors related to CVD risk that are amenable to change (e.g., diet, physical activity, smoking), in contrast to those that are intrinsic to the individual (e.g., age, sex, race, genetic traits).

mortality: rate of death expressed as the number of deaths occurring in a population of given size within a specified time interval (e.g., 265 annual deaths from heart disease per 100,000 U.S. Hispanic women, 1991–1995).

obesity: usually defined in terms of body mass index (BMI), which is calculated as body weight in kilograms (1 kg = 2.2 lbs) divided by height in meters (1 m = 39.37 in) squared; adults with a BMI of ≥30.0 kg/m^2 are considered "obese," and those with a BMI of 25–29.9 kg/m^2 are considered "overweight." In children, overweight is defined as BMI greater than the 95th percentile value for the same age and sex group.

overt disease: for CVD, disease with signs or symptoms that are recognizable by the affected individual or health care provider.

overweight: see *obesity*.

peripheral arteries: arteries in the upper and lower extremities (arms and legs).

peripheral arterial disease: mainly atherosclerosis of the extremities; especially important in the lower extremities; also called peripheral vascular disease.

physical inactivity: lack of habitual activity sufficient to maintain good health, resulting in an unfavorable balance between energy intake and expenditure and fostering the development of overweight or obesity and other risk factors for heart disease and stroke.

plaque: the characteristic manifestation of atherosclerosis located in the arterial wall and extending into the lumen or channel of the artery; plaque can disturb or restrict blood flow and is prone to fissure or rupture, thus precipitating formation of blood clots that can cause an acute coronary event.

policy and environmental change: an intervention approach to reducing the burden of chronic diseases that focuses on enacting effective policies (e.g., laws, regulations, formal and informal rules) or promoting environmental change (e.g., changes to economic, social, or physical environments).

population-based observations: health data that pertain to a defined, usually large, population (e.g., vital statistics, surveillance, results of population surveys).

population-wide approach: an intervention strategy that targets the population as a whole without regard to the risk levels of various subgroups; distinguished from and complementary to the *high-risk approach*.

prevalence: the frequency of a particular condition within a defined population at a designated time (e.g., 12.6 million Americans living with heart disease in 1999 or 36.4% of African American men aged 20–74 years found to have hypertension in a survey conducted in 1988–1994).

prevention research: aims to prevent disease and promote health by developing and disseminating strategies applicable to public health programs and policies.

preventive dose: the intensity and duration of appropriate public health interventions needed to achieve their goals; similar to the dose and duration of medical treatment sufficient to control or cure an illness.

primary CVD prevention: a set of interventions, including the detection and control of risk factors, designed to prevent the first occurrence of heart attack, heart failure, or stroke among people with identifiable risk factors; this approach corresponds most directly to the objectives of goal 2 for preventing heart disease and stroke of the Healthy People 2010 Heart and Stroke Partnership.

primordial CVD prevention: a set of interventions targeting people without risk factors or CVD (including the maintenance or restoration of favorable social and environmental conditions and the promotion of healthy behavioral patterns) to prevent development of risk factors; this approach corresponds most directly to the objectives of goal 1 for preventing heart disease and stroke of the Healthy People 2010 Heart and Stroke Partnership. Although this approach was originally intended to apply to whole societies to prevent the first appearance of epidemic levels of risk factors, the term is commonly used in the sense of "early intervention" to prevent risk factors in individuals even in populations where risk factors are already epidemic; in the *Action Plan*, "CVH promotion" is used as equivalent to "primordial prevention."

priority populations: groups at especially high risk for CVD (e.g., those identified by sex, race or ethnicity, education, income, disability, place of residence, or sexual orientation).

randomized controlled trial: an experimental study of an intervention, most often a medical treatment, in which study participants are randomly assigned to treatment or comparison groups; much less often, communities rather than individuals are the units used to form treatment and comparison groups.

rehabilitation: an intervention approach designed to limit disability among survivors of CVD events and reduce their risk for subsequent events.

risk behavior: a behavioral pattern associated with increased frequency of specified health problems; for example, high salt intake, smoking, and binge drinking are all associated with CVD.

risk factor: an individual characteristic associated with increased frequency of specified health problems; for example, high LDL cholesterol, high blood pressure, and diabetes are all associated with CVD.

risk factor detection and control: an intervention approach that targets people with identifiable risk factors; includes both screening or other methods of detection and long-term disease management through changes in lifestyle, behavior, medication (when necessary).

secondary CVD prevention: a set of interventions aimed at survivors of acute CVD events (e.g., heart attack, heart failure, stroke) or others with known CVD in which long-term case management is used to reduce disability and risk for subsequent CVD events; this approach corresponds most directly to the objectives of goal 4 for preventing heart disease and stroke of the Healthy People 2010 Heart and Stroke Partnership.

stroke: sudden interruption of blood supply to the brain caused by an obstruction or the rupture of a blood vessel.

subclinical disease: presence of one or more forms of CVD (e.g., atherosclerosis, coronary heart disease) detectable only by special examination (e.g., ankle-arm blood pressure ratio, carotid artery ultrasound examination, electrocardiogram) and not recognizable from signs or symptoms expressed by the affected person.

survival: remaining alive for a specified period (e.g., beyond the 28-day definition of case fatality) after a CVD event.

tertiary CVD prevention: an intervention approach included in secondary prevention, as it is used in the *Action Plan*; sometimes distinguished as reducing disability among survivors of CVD events through rehabilitation; this approach combined with secondary prevention corresponds most directly to the objectives of goal 4 for preventing heart disease and stroke of the Healthy People 2010 Heart and Stroke Partnership.

vascular cognitive impairment: loss of mental function that occurs in association with a stroke, sometimes followed by dementia.

APPENDIX B: NATIONAL GOALS AND OBJECTIVES

The matrix in this appendix matches the *Healthy People 2010* objectives most pertinent to heart disease and stroke with the four goals identified by the Healthy People 2010 Heart and Stroke Partnership. These goals are based on Chapter 12, Heart Disease and Stroke, of *Healthy People 2010*. In addition to the 16 objectives listed in this chapter, 48 objectives in other chapters could, if addressed, help to achieve the four goals.

		Goal 1	Goal 2	Goal 3	Goal 4
		Prevention of risk factors	Detection and treatment of risk factors	Early detection and treatment of heart attacks and strokes	Prevention of recurrent cardiovascular events
Objectives from Chapter 12, Heart Disease and Stroke					
12-1	Coronary heart disease (CHD) deaths	X	X	X	X
12-2	Knowledge of symptoms of heart attack and importance of calling 911 (D*)			X	
12-3	Artery-opening therapy (D)			X	
12-4	Bystander response to cardiac arrest (D)			X	
12-5	Out-of-hospital emergency care (D)			X	
12-6	Heart failure hospitalizations				X
12-7	Stroke deaths	X	X	X	X
12-8	Knowledge of early warning symptoms of stroke (D)			X	X
12-9	High blood pressure	X	X		X
12-10	High blood pressure control		X		X
12-11	Action to help control blood pressure		X		X
12-12	Blood pressure monitoring	X	X		
12-13	Mean total blood cholesterol levels	X	X		X
12-14	High blood cholesterol levels	X	X		X
12-15	Blood cholesterol screening	X	X		X
12-16	LDL-cholesterol level in CHD patients (D)				X
Objectives from Chapter 1, Access to Quality Health Services					
1-3	Counseling about health behaviors	X	X	X	X
1-7	Core competencies in health provider training (D)	X	X	X	X
1-10	Delay or difficulty in getting emergency care (D)			X	
1-11	Rapid prehospital emergency care (D)			X	
Objectives from Chapter 4, Chronic Kidney Disease					
4-2	Cardiovascular (CVD) deaths in persons with chronic kidney failure			X	X
Objectives from Chapter 5, Diabetes					
5-2	New cases of diabetes	X			
5-4	Prevent diabetes	X			
5-7	Cardiovascular deaths in persons with diabetes	X	X		X
Objectives from Chapter 7, Educational and Community-Based Programs					
7-2	School health education	X	X	X	X
7-5	Worksite health promotion programs	X	X	X	X
7-8	Satisfaction with patient education (D)	X	X	X	X
7-10	Community health promotion programs (D)	X	X	X	X
7-11	Culturally appropriate community health promotion	X	X	X	X
7-12	Older adult participation in community health promotion activities	X	X	X	X

	Goal 1 **Prevention of risk factors**	Goal 2 **Detection and treatment of risk factors**	Goal 3 **Early detection and treatment of heart attacks and strokes**	Goal 4 **Prevention of recurrent cardiovascular events**
Objectives from Chapter 11, Health Communication				
11-1 Households with Internet access	X	X	X	X
11-2 Health literacy (D)	X			
11-4 Quality of Internet health information sources	X	X	X	X
11-6 Satisfaction with providers' communication skills (D)	X	X	X	X
Objectives from Chapter 19, Nutrition and Overweight				
19-1 Healthy weight in adults	X			X
19-2 Obesity in adults	X	X		X
19-3 Overweight or obesity in children and adolescents	X	X		
19-5 Fruit intake	X			
19-6 Vegetable intake	X			
19-8 Saturated fat intake	X			
19-9 Total fat intake	X			
19-11 Calcium intake	X			
19-16 Worksite promotion of nutrition education and weight management	X	X	X	X
Objectives from Chapter 22, Physical Activity and Fitness				
22-1 No leisure-time physical activity	X			X
22-2 Moderate physical activity	X			X
22-3 Vigorous physical activity	X			X
22-6 Moderate physical activity in adolescents	X			
22-7 Vigorous physical activity in adolescents	X			
22-11 Television viewing	X			
22-13 Worksite physical activity and fitness	X			X
22-14 Community walking	X			X
22-15 Community bicycling	X			X
Objectives from Chapter 23, Public Health Infrastructure				
23-1 Public health employee access to Internet (D)	X	X	X	X
23-3 Use of geocoding in health data systems	X	X	X	X
23-10 Continuing education and training by public health agencies (D)	X	X	X	X
23-16 Data on public health expenditures (D)	X	X	X	X
Objectives from Chapter 27, Tobacco Use				
27-1 Adult tobacco use	X			X
27-2 Adolescent tobacco use	X			
27-3 Initiation of tobacco use (D)	X	X	X	X
27-4 Age at first use of tobacco	X			
27-5 Smoking cessation by adults	X	X		X
27-10 Exposure to environmental tobacco smoke	X			
27-16 Tobacco advertising and promotion targeting adolescents and young adults (D)	X	X	X	X
27-17 Adolescent disapproval of smoking	X	X	X	X

* Developmental (D) objectives provide a vision for a desired outcome or health status. All other objectives are considered measurable objectives, which provide direction for action.

Source: US Department of Health and Human Services. *Healthy People 2010: Understanding and Improving Health and Objectives for Improving Health.* 2nd ed. 2 vols. Washington, DC: US Government Printing Office; November 2000.

APPENDIX C: PROFILES OF THE CO-LEAD AGENCIES FOR THE *HEALTHY PEOPLE 2010* HEART DISEASE AND STROKE FOCUS AREA

The Centers for Disease Control and Prevention and the National Institutes of Health are co-lead federal agencies responsible for undertaking activities to move the nation toward achieving the *Healthy People 2010* goal for preventing heart disease and stroke and for reporting progress on the objectives for this focus area over the next decade. The following profiles highlight the work of these agencies in heart disease and stroke prevention. An exhaustive account of these and related activities is beyond the scope of this document, but further details and updates can be obtained from each agency's Web site.

Centers for Disease Control and Prevention (CDC)
www.cdc.gov

CDC is recognized as the lead federal agency for protecting the health and safety of people at home and abroad, providing credible information to enhance health decisions, and promoting health through strong partnerships. CDC serves as the national focus for developing and applying disease prevention and control, environmental health, and health promotion and education activities designed to improve the health of the people of the United States.

National Center for Chronic Disease Prevention and Health Promotion

CDC's National Center for Chronic Disease Prevention and Health Promotion (NCCD-PHP) is at the forefront of the nation's efforts to prevent and control chronic diseases. The center conducts studies to better understand the causes of chronic diseases, supports programs to promote healthy behaviors, and monitors the health of the nation through surveys. Critical to the success of these efforts are partnerships with state health and education agencies, voluntary associations, private organizations, and other federal agencies. Together, the center and its partners are working to create a healthier nation.

Chronic diseases—such as heart disease, cancer, and diabetes—are the leading causes of death and disability in the United States. These diseases account for 7 of every 10 deaths and affect the quality of life of 90 million Americans. Although chronic diseases are among the most common and costly health problems, they are also among the most preventable. Adopting healthy behaviors such as eating nutritious foods, being physically active, and avoiding tobacco use can prevent or control the devastating effects of these diseases.

In the area of cardiovascular health (CVH), the center established in October 2000 the Cardiovascular Health Coordinating Committee, whose primary responsibility is communication and coordination among the several NCCDPHP divisions most actively engaged in CVH: the Divisions of Adult and Community Health, Adolescent and School Health, Diabetes Translation, and Nutrition and Physical Activity and the Office on Smoking and Health. Highlights of relevant programs in these divisions are outlined in the following sections.

State Heart Disease and Stroke Prevention Program

In 1998, Congress funded CDC to launch a nationwide effort to help states develop the capacity, commitment, and resources necessary for a comprehensive program to prevent death and disability from heart disease and stroke and to improve the cardiovascular health of all Americans. CDC funds states for basic implementation or at a lower capacity-building level. Program priorities include the following:

- Prevent and control high blood pressure and high blood cholesterol levels.
- Improve quality of care to prevent and manage high blood pressure, stroke, and heart disease.
- Get people to appropriate emergency care quickly.
- Eliminate health disparities (e.g., based on geography, gender, race or ethnicity, or income).
- Promote heart health in a variety of settings (health care facilities, work sites, schools, and communities) through education and policy and environmental changes.

CDC works with partners both inside and beyond the health sector to address the *Healthy People 2010* objectives for preventing heart disease and stroke. Partners include other federal agencies (e.g., Centers for Medicare & Medicaid Services, National Institutes of Health), national health organizations (e.g., American Heart Association/American Stroke Association, National Stroke Association), and professional groups (e.g., American College of Cardiology).

Surveillance of Heart Disease and Stroke

As part of its national leadership, CDC supports and conducts the surveillance necessary to build a strong foundation of science for preventing heart disease and stroke. The resulting data can be used to guide state and local public health programs. For example, the recently released *Atlas of Stroke Mortality: Racial, Ethnic and Geographic Disparities in the United States* presents detailed national and state maps with county-level data of local disparities in heart disease and stroke death rates for the nation's five largest racial and ethnic groups. This publication is the third in a series on cardiovascular health, following *Women and Heart Disease: An Atlas of Racial and Ethnic Disparities in Mortality* and *Men and Heart Disease: An Atlas of Racial and Ethnic Disparities in Mortality*.

In 2001, CDC established the Paul Coverdell National Acute Stroke Registry to design and test prototypes to measure the delivery of acute care for stroke. Eight sites are developing prototypes for statewide, hospital-based registries that are expected to improve hospitals' delivery of the critical emergency care that can prevent permanent disabilities from stroke.

Prevention Research Centers (PRCs) Program

In 1984, Congress authorized the secretary of the U.S. Department of Health and Human Services (HHS) to create a network of academic health centers to conduct applied public health research. The first three centers were funded two years later. CDC was selected to administer the PRC network and to provide leadership, technical assistance, and oversight.

Individual behaviors and environmental factors cause many chronic diseases as well as injuries and some infections. Prevention researchers develop strategies to help people reduce risk factors in their lives and their communities. By involving community members, academic researchers, and public health agencies, the PRCs find innovative ways to promote health and prevent disease. Together, these partners design, test, and disseminate strategies—often as new policies or recommended public health practices.

PRCs are associated with schools of public health, medicine, or osteopathy and are located throughout the country. Each center conducts at least one core research project with an underserved population that has a disproportionately large burden of disease and disability. The centers also work with partners on special interest projects defined by CDC and other HHS agencies. Expertise gained from this work makes the centers competitive for research funding from other sources.

PRCs are a national resource for developing effective prevention strategies and applying those strategies at the community level. Each center encourages interaction among faculty from different disciplines (e.g., education, social work, psychology, nursing), whose expertise is essential to solving complex health and psychosocial problems.

Behavioral Risk Factor Surveillance System (BRFSS)

The BRFSS is a state-based system of health surveys established in 1984 by CDC. Information on health risk behaviors, clinical preventive health practices, and health care access, primarily related to chronic disease and injury, is obtained from a representative sample of adults in each state. For most states, the BRFSS is the only source for this type of information. Currently, data are collected monthly in all 50 states, the District of Columbia, and Puerto Rico; annual point-in-time surveys are conducted in the Virgin Islands and Guam. Interviews are completed each year with more than 200,000 adults, making the BRFSS the largest telephone health survey in the world. In addition to being a unique source of risk behavior data for states, the BRFSS is also useful for measuring progress toward *Healthy People 2010* national objectives. Seven of the 10 leading health indicators for 2010 can be assessed through the BRFSS.

As the demand for data has increased, so has the number of requests to add questions to the survey. Currently, almost every division in NCCDPHP and other CDC Centers, Institutes, and Offices has questions on the BRFSS. Interest in the BRFSS has also grown outside CDC. Other federal agencies, such as the Health Resources and Services Administration (HRSA), the Administration on Aging (AoA), and the Department of Veterans Affairs (VA), have added questions. Requests for technical assistance also have come from other countries that are eager to develop similar surveillance systems, notably China, Australia, Canada, and Russia. The World Health Organization (WHO) is developing a model surveillance system based on the BRFSS for export to any country.

As the BRFSS data have become more useful, the demand for more local data (i.e., district-, county-, or city-level data) has increased. This demand led to the Selected Cities Project, in which data from the 1997–2000 BRFSS were used to calculate estimates for selected urban areas in the United States with at least 300 respondents. This project has yielded estimates for nearly 200 metropolitan areas for the 1997–1999 combined data. The 2000 data provided estimates for 100 metropolitan areas. Preliminary results showed that the prevalence of certain behaviors varied across cities, not unlike the differences found across states. Variation in prevalence was also observed when cities were compared with their surrounding metropolitan areas and with the rest of the state. Plans are to add the new weights soon to the BRFSS public-use data file, allowing researchers outside CDC to analyze data for metropolitan areas. This new use of BRFSS data fills a critical public health need for local surveillance data to support targeted program implementation and evaluation, and these data should help cities to better plan and direct their prevention efforts.

Racial and Ethnic Approaches to Community Health (REACH) 2010

REACH 2010 is the cornerstone of CDC's efforts to eliminate racial and ethnic disparities in health, one of the two overarching goals of *Healthy People 2010*. Launched in 1999, REACH 2010 is designed to eliminate disparities in the following six priority areas: cardiovascular disease, immunizations, breast and cervical cancer screening and management, diabetes, HIV infections/AIDS, and infant mortality. The racial and ethnic groups targeted are African Americans, American Indians, Alaska Natives, Asian Americans, Hispanic Americans, and Pacific Islanders.

REACH 2010 is a two-phase, 5-year demonstration project that supports community coalitions in designing, implementing, and evaluating community-driven strategies to eliminate health disparities. Each coalition comprises a community-based organization and three other organizations, of which at least one is either a local or state health department or a university or research group.

During a 12-month planning phase, REACH 2010 grantees use local data to develop a community action plan that addresses one or more of the six priority areas and targets one or more racial and ethnic minority groups. During the 4-year implementation phase, community coalitions carry out activities outlined in their community action plans and evaluate program activities.

Evaluating REACH 2010 programs is critically important in determining their effectiveness in reducing health disparities. Working with its grantees and partners, CDC has developed an evaluation model to guide the collection of national data. This model evaluates programs on their effectiveness in the following areas: building community capacity, developing targeted actions, improving health systems and agents of change, decreasing risk behaviors and increasing protective behaviors, and reducing disparity-related illness and death.

REACH 2010 projects are empowering community members to transform their neighborhoods into places that encourage people to adopt and sustain healthy behaviors and to avoid risk behaviors. Through close collaboration with community members and creative partnerships with public and private organizations, CDC will continue to spearhead the country's efforts to eliminate health disparities by carrying out the lessons learned from the REACH 2010 projects in communities across the country.

School Health

Every school day, 53 million young people attend nearly 117,000 schools across our nation. Because of the size and accessibility of this population, school health programs are one of the most efficient means to reach young people and prevent/address behaviors that lead to serious health problems. CDC began an initiative in 1992 to support coordinated school health programs in the states that promote healthy behavior, such as eating nutritious foods, being physically active, and avoiding tobacco use. These programs aim to reduce young people's risk for developing chronic diseases later in life.

CDC funding and assistance enable state departments of education and health to work together efficiently, respond to changing health priorities, and use limited resources effectively to meet a wide range of health needs among the state's school-aged population.

CDC has also established a national framework to support these programs. More than 40 national, nongovernmental education and health organizations work with CDC to develop model policies, guidelines, and training to help states establish high-quality school health programs. Through this national framework and in collaboration with health and education partners, CDC helps funded states provide young people with information and skills needed to choose healthy behaviors. The eight components of a coordinated school health program include health education, nutrition services, physical education, health services, health promotion for staff, counseling and psychological services, a healthy school environment, and parent and community involvement.

Since 1991, the Youth Risk Behavior Surveillance System (YRBSS) has provided data on health-related behaviors, such as tobacco use, physical activity levels, and fruit and vegetable intake, among young people. Developed by CDC with federal, state, and private-sector partners, this voluntary system includes a national survey of high school students plus surveys conducted by state and local education and health agencies. The YRBSS provides vital information to improve health programs.

Because national efforts for coordinated school health programs have been hampered by a lack of information on school health policies and programs, CDC has conducted the School Health Policies and Programs Study (SHPPS). SHPPS provides valuable answers to questions about programs in areas such as health education, physical education, and school food service at state, district, school, and classroom levels.

To help schools plan and implement effective health policies and programs, CDC has published guidelines for school health programs. These guidelines are based on a synthesis of theory, research, and best practices and were developed jointly by scientific experts, school practitioners, and appropriate national organizations. To help schools implement these guidelines, CDC has developed several tools, including *The School Health Index: A Self-Assessment and Planning Guide*, and supported development of other tools, such as *Fit, Healthy, and Ready to Learn: A School Health Policy Guide*, which was produced by the National Association of State Boards of Education.

Diabetes Prevention and Control

CDC provides leadership and funding to diabetes prevention and control programs nationwide. CDC also works with many partners to provide data for sound public health decisions, inform the public about diabetes, and ensure good care and education for Americans with diabetes. CDC provides support to states, territories, and the District of Columbia for core diabetes control programs and more substantial support to some states for comprehensive programs.

Timely data and public health research are essential for understanding how diabetes affects different populations and for improving quality of care. CDC analyzes information from several national data sources, including the BRFSS, and explores ways to collect better diabetes data on groups most at risk. To translate scientific data into higher-quality care, CDC works with many research partners, including the National Diabetes Laboratory. CDC also works with managed care organizations and community health centers to
- Assess how accepted standards of diabetes care are applied by health care providers and in clinical care settings.
- Explore variations in the quality of diabetes care provided.
- Develop and test strategies to move existing care practices closer to optimal standards.

Educating others about diabetes is a priority at CDC. The National Diabetes Education Program (NDEP) has a network of more than 200 public and private partners that provide education to improve treatment, promote early detection, and prevent the onset of diabetes. The NDEP is sponsored by CDC and the National Institutes of Health, and many NDEP products are available on the Internet (www.ndep.nih.gov).

CDC also develops new resources for health professionals, people with diabetes, and communities, including Diabetes Today, a train-the-trainer program that allows health professionals and community leaders to develop a community plan for preventing the complications of diabetes.

Nutrition and Physical Activity

Beginning in fiscal year 2001, Congress appropriated funds that allow CDC to help states plan and initiate nutrition and physical activity programs to help prevent and control obesity and other chronic diseases. With further funding, CDC will help to expand these programs and will support research to increase physical activity and improve nutrition in states and communities.

In 1995, CDC's landmark publication, *Physical Activity and Health: A Report of the Surgeon General*, brought together the results of decades of research on physical activity and health. Among its findings were that physical activity need not be strenuous to produce benefits and that inactive people can improve their health by becoming moderately active on a regular basis. The implications of these findings compel CDC to ensure that physical activity receives the attention and commitment given to other important public health issues. CDC research is strengthening knowledge of the role of physical activity and nutrition in health.

To further address these issues, CDC has established a nationwide framework for coordinated health education programs in schools. Inactivity and unhealthy diets are among the risk behaviors that these programs address. CDC has also collaborated with national health and education organizations to develop guidelines and materials to help schools promote healthy eating and physical activity.

Since the 1950s, the infrastructure to support walking and bicycling in the United States has been neglected. Trips made by walking or cycling have declined by more than 40% since 1977. CDC's Active Community Environments Initiative (ACES) works with partners to promote the development of accessible recreation facilities, including more opportunities for walking and cycling.

The National 5-A-Day program, which is a comprehensive, coordinated national nutrition program designed to increase consumption of fruits and vegetables to five or more servings each day by the year 2010, is implementing recommendations from a recent comprehensive review. The most significant recommendations were to strengthen and expand the program's organizational structure to include new partners and to support research, surveillance, and applied public health programs to increase vegetable and fruit consumption. The National Cancer Institute, the U.S. Department of Agriculture, and CDC are currently defining the roles and responsibilities of each partner in the new model.

Well-Integrated Screening and Evaluation for Women Across the Nation (WISEWOMAN)

WISEWOMAN is a CDC-funded program that helps women in need gain access to screening and lifestyle interventions that can reduce their risk for heart disease and other chronic diseases. Eligible women are 40–64 years old and have little or no health insurance. Many are from racial and ethnic minority populations. WISEWOMAN is the result of 1993 legislation that expanded the services offered within the National Breast and Cervical Cancer Early Detection Program (NBCCEDP). Through the NBCCEDP, CDC helps states, territories, and tribal organizations provide potentially life-saving screening for breast and cervical cancers to low-income and uninsured women. Through WISEWOMAN projects and community partnerships, women participating in the NBCCEDP are offered screenings and interventions for obesity, sedentary behavior, poor dietary habits, high blood pressure, high cholesterol, and smoking. Some projects also screen women for diabetes or osteoporosis, because these conditions also are affected by nutrition and physical activity. WISEWOMAN staff also provide referrals when treatment is needed.

Smoking and Health

CDC provides national leadership for a comprehensive, broad-based approach to reducing tobacco use. A variety of federal, state, and local government agencies; professional and voluntary organizations; and academic institutions have joined together to advance this comprehensive approach, which involves

- Preventing young people from starting to smoke.
- Eliminating exposure to secondhand smoke.
- Promoting quitting.
- Identifying and eliminating disparities in tobacco use among different population groups.

Essential elements of this approach include state- and community-based interventions, countermarketing, policy development, surveillance, and evaluation. These activities target groups (e.g., young people, racial and ethnic minority groups, people with low incomes or low levels of education, and women) at highest risk for tobacco-related health problems.

CDC supports programs to prevent and control tobacco use in all 50 states, 7 territories, 7 tribal organizations, and the District of Columbia. Supplemental funding is provided to some programs to identify tobacco-related disparities and develop strategic plans for reducing them. CDC also funds national networks to promote prevention and control efforts among organizations that serve priority populations; provides grants to states for coordinated school health programs that include components for preventing tobacco use; and provides technical assistance to help states plan, establish, and evaluate tobacco control programs.

CDC recently released several publications to help states manage their tobacco control programs, including *Best Practices for Comprehensive Tobacco Control Programs, Reducing Tobacco Use: A Report of the Surgeon General, and Investment in Tobacco Control: State Highlights 2002.* Guidance is also offered through CDC's *Guidelines for School Health Programs to Prevent Tobacco Use and Addiction* and the *Guide to Community Preventive Services: Tobacco Use Prevention and Control.*

To strengthen the scientific foundation for preventing and controlling tobacco use, CDC examines trends, health effects, and economic costs. Examples include the U.S. Surgeon General's reports on the health consequences of tobacco use, published since 1964; CDC's air toxicants laboratory, which is developing and applying laboratory technology to prevent death and disease from tobacco use and exposure to secondhand smoke; and the school-based Global Youth Tobacco Survey (GYTS), developed by WHO and CDC to track tobacco use among young people in over 140 countries using a common methodology and a core questionnaire. In addition, CDC's National Tobacco Information Online System (NATIONS) provides country-level data on tobacco use and its health effects, laws and regulations, and economics, and CDC's State Tobacco Activities Tracking and Evaluation (STATE) System provides similar state-level data.

CDC researches, develops, and distributes tobacco and health information nationwide. It also distributes hundreds of thousands of publications and video products each year and provides information and databases through its Web site. Through its Media Campaign Resource Center and its interactive database, CDC provides high-quality counteradvertising materials and technical assistance to help state and local programs conduct media campaigns to prevent tobacco use.

CDC's health communication messages continue to focus on reducing smoking among young people while increasing the emphasis on helping people to quit, reducing exposure to secondhand smoke, and reducing disparities. In partnership with other federal, state, and local agencies, CDC communicates key tobacco messages through the media, schools, and communities.

As the only WHO Collaborating Center on Global Tobacco Prevention and Control in North America, CDC implements international studies, conducts epidemiologic research, and provides international assistance on reducing tobacco use.

National Center for Environmental Health (NCEH)

The National Center for Environmental Health (NCEH) is dedicated to serving the global community by providing leadership, through science and service, to promote health and quality of life by preventing and controlling disease, disability, and death resulting from interactions between people and their environment. NCEH activities most directly related to CVH include laboratory programs, such as the Lipid Standardization Program, and the Public Health Genomics Program.

Lipid Standardization Program (LSP)

CDC developed and maintains reference methods and serum-based reference materials for total cholesterol (TC), high-density lipoprotein cholesterol (HDLC), low-density lipoprotein cholesterol (LDLC), and triglycerides (TG). In 1957, CDC began efforts to standardize cholesterol measurement and became the first to develop a standardization program designed to improve and normalize clinical test results. In 1961, CDC, in collaboration with the National Heart, Lung, and Blood Institute (NHLBI), National Institutes of Health, developed and continues to maintain a three-phase LSP to provide an accuracy-based standard for measuring TC, HDLC, LDLC, and TG in national and international lipid laboratories.

The LSP's standardization efforts extend to a variety of clinical trials and population studies, including the
- Multiple Risk Factor Intervention Trial (MRFIT).
- Framingham Heart Study.
- Lipid Research Clinics-Coronary Primary Prevention Trial (LRC-CPPT).
- Women's Health Initiative.

- West of Scotland Coronary Prevention Study (WOSCOPS).
- Air Force/Texas Coronary Atherosclerosis Prevention Study (AFCAPS/TexCAPS).
- National Health and Nutrition Examination Surveys (NHANES).

Each year, about 100 domestic and international laboratories participate in the LSP and receive about 16,000 individual vials of fresh-frozen serum reference samples to assess laboratory performance.

As a result of frequent and responsive assessments of laboratory performance, CDC ensures the accuracy and uniformity of population-study and clinical-trial data, regardless of the testing method or the analytical system used. These clinical investigations provide cardiovascular medicine with a reliable scientific database for evaluating risk factors associated with CVD. This database provides the basis for the National Cholesterol Education Program's (NCEP's) intervention strategy to reduce morbidity and mortality from CVD. CDC's Lipid Reference Laboratory is the cornerstone of the National Reference System for Cholesterol to which all cholesterol measurements are traceable, thus ensuring reliable testing results in the nation's clinical laboratories.

Cholesterol Reference Method Laboratory Network (CRMLN)

CDC established the CRMLN to help manufacturers calibrate diagnostic products used for lipid and lipoprotein testing. CDC researchers believe that working with manufacturers is the most effective way to improve and standardize these measurements within clinical laboratories and to achieve the NCEP's goals. CRMLN laboratories use CDC reference methods or designated comparison methods (DCMs) that are closely linked to CDC reference methods. Manufacturer certification is based on the analysis of fresh samples from patients by both the diagnostic test method and the CRMLN laboratory. Manufacturers who successfully complete the comparison are issued a Certificate of Traceability, which is valid for two years. Manufacturers are encouraged to repeat the certification on a regular basis. This approach ensures that diagnostic products are properly calibrated and traceable to the accuracy base maintained by CDC.

C-Reactive Protein Standardization Program

CDC convened a forum for manufacturers of high sensitive C-reactive protein (hs-CRP) assays to identify measurement problems, discuss the need for developing a reference method and materials, and plan approaches for methodology improvement and standardization. CDC conducted a major study to evaluate various materials for their applicability and commutability as potential reference materials for calibration and standardization of hs-CRP. CDC co-sponsored with NHLBI, the American College of Cardiology, the American Heart Association, and the American Association for Clinical Chemistry a special focus workshop to address issues concerning the appropriate clinical use of hs-CRP in predicting risk for CVD. This led to publication in 2003 of the American Heart Association/CDC Scientific Statement, *Markers of Inflammation and Cardiovascular Diseases: Application to Clinical and Public Health Practice.* CDC is helping the College of American Pathologists (CAP) implement proficiency testing surveys for hs-CRP and Lp(a) as part of its efforts to establish a cardiac risk survey program.

Homocysteine Standardization Program

CDC is addressing the need for accurate and precise laboratory measurements of plasma homocysteine on many fronts. Using a CDC reference method, the laboratory measures plasma homocysteine levels in samples obtained from participants in the NHANES. In 1998, CDC conducted an international laboratory comparison study for plasma homocysteine with 14 laboratories to evaluate method differences. In 2000, CDC helped the CAP develop its first homocysteine survey. CDC continues to provide confirmation values for each CAP homocysteine survey on the basis of results obtained using the CDC reference method. CDC is collaborating with the Mayo Clinic to evaluate a mass spectrometry method that the Mayo Clinic developed as a potential high-order reference method. CDC is also collaborating with the National Institute of Standards and Technologies to support reference materials development. CDC participates in the International Federation of Clinical Chemistry Working Group for Homocysteine Standardization. CDC continuously evaluates new assays for measuring homocysteine and publishes evaluation results in professional journals.

Genomics and Disease Prevention

To move beyond gene discovery to public health action requires additional research and planning. Clinical and epidemiologic studies are needed to assess the interaction between genetics and environment in causing disease and to evaluate the clinical validity and utility of genetic tests. Public health policies are needed to address related social, ethical, and legal issues and to guarantee access to genetic services. Training the public health workforce and keeping the public informed are also important components of a plan to integrate genetics into public health. CDC's activities in genomics and disease prevention reflect the enormity of the challenge facing public health today. They are based on a commitment to meet the challenge to use genetic information to improve health and prevent disease in the 21st century.

In October 2001, CDC established Centers for Genomics and Public Health in schools of public health at the Universities of Michigan, North Carolina, and Washington. The centers will help build the knowledge base on genomics and public health, focusing on chronic diseases with modifiable environmental risk factors such as diet, exercise, or exposure to chemicals. They will also provide training and technical assistance to local, state, and regional public health organizations. The Center at the University of Michigan is focused on cardiovascular diseases.

In collaboration with CDC, the Chronic Disease Directors convened a Genomics and Chronic Disease Summit in Atlanta in early 2002 to focus on emerging human genetic information relevant to prevention of cardiovascular disease, as well as asthma, cancer, diabetes, and obesity.

CDC is evaluating family history as a tool for assessing risk and influencing early detection and prevention of common diseases, including coronary heart disease, stroke, and hypertension. Coordinated by CDC's Office of Genomics and Disease Prevention (OGDP), this collaborative effort includes several CDC programs and NIH institutes, including CDC's Cardiovascular Health Branch and NHLBI, respectively.

A CDC-wide working group has developed a proposal for analyzing DNA samples collected in the NHANES III to determine the prevalence of genotypes of potential public health importance in a nationally representative, population-based sample and demographic subgroups. The proposal encompasses genes in pathways considered important in the pathogenesis and progression of cardiovascular diseases, including folate and homocysteine metabolism, lipid metabolism, blood pressure regulation, and hemostasis.

Epidemiological research is needed to understand how modifiable risk factors (e.g., diet, chemical exposures, infections, lifestyle) interact with genetic factors in the causation and progression of cardiovascular disease and to suggest ways that this information can help target disease prevention efforts. Through the 1999 Prevention Research Initiative, CDC funded the University of Texas Houston Health Science Center to study gene-environment interactions related to cardiovascular disease in over 15,000 African American and white men and women aged 45–64 years who participated in the multicenter Arteriosclerosis Risk in Communities (ARIC) Study conducted by NHLBI.

CDC supports the Stroke Prevention in Young Women Study, a population-based case-control study in Maryland and the District of Columbia that seeks to identify behavioral and genetic factors that may help explain the increased risk for stroke among African American women. CDC funds the Oregon Sudden Unexplained Death Study, which tracks all cardiac arrests that occur in Multnomah County, Oregon, and assesses the determinants of sudden death.

National Center for Health Statistics (NCHS)

As the nation's principal health statistics agency, NCHS compiles statistical information to guide actions and policies to improve the health of our people. NCHS is a unique public resource for health information—a critical element of public health and health policy. NCHS health statistics are used to

- Document the health status of the population and of important subgroups.
- Identify disparities in health status and use of health care by race, ethnicity, socioeconomic status, region, and other population gradients.
- Describe people's experiences with the health care system.
- Monitor trends in health status and health care delivery.
- Identify health problems.
- Support biomedical and health services research.
- Provide information for making changes in public policies and programs.
- Evaluate the impact of health policies and programs.

Working with partners throughout the health community, NCHS uses a variety of approaches to efficiently obtain information from the sources most able to provide information. The center collects data from birth and death records, medical records, interview surveys, and through direct physical exams and laboratory testing. NCHS is a key element of our national public health infrastructure, providing important surveillance information that helps identify and address critical health problems.

NCHS employs a variety of data collection mechanisms to obtain accurate information from multiple sources. This process provides multiple perspectives to help understand the population's health, influences on health, and health outcomes.

National Vital Statistics System (NVSS)

The NVSS provides the nation's official vital statistics data on the basis of the collection and registration of birth and death events at the state and local level. The NVSS provides the most complete and continuous data available to public health officials at the national, state, and local levels and in the private sector. Vital statistics are a critical component of our national health information system, allowing us to monitor progress toward achieving health and welfare reform goals.

Examples of NVSS data include
- Number of teen births.
- Prenatal care and birthweight.
- Risk factors for adverse pregnancy outcomes.
- Firearm-related mortality in teens.
- Infant mortality rates.
- Leading causes of death.
- Life expectancy.
- Firearm-related mortality.

National Health Care Survey (NHCS)

The NHCS is a family of surveys that collects data from health care establishments about the use of services across the major sectors of the U.S. health care system. These data may be used to profile changes in the use of health care resources, patterns of disease, and the impact of new medications and technologies. Information on the characteristics of providers, facilities, and patients allows researchers to study shifts in the delivery of care across the health care system, variations in treatment patterns, and patient outcomes.

Provider sites surveyed include
- Hospitals.
- Nursing homes.
- Emergency departments.
- Hospital outpatient departments.
- Office-based physicians.
- Ambulatory surgery centers.
- Home health agencies.
- Hospices.

National Health and Nutrition Examination Survey (NHANES)

The NHANES is NCHS's most in-depth and logistically complex survey, designed to assess the health and nutritional status of Americans. This comprehensive survey combines personal interviews with standardized physical and dental examinations, diagnostic procedures, and lab tests for approximately 5,000 persons each year.

The survey provides information related to
- Diseases.
- Health risk factors.
- Genetics and health.
- Diet and nutritional health status.
- Oral health.
- Environmental exposures.
- Obesity and physical fitness.

National Health Interview Survey (NHIS)

The NHIS provides information annually on the health status of the U.S. civilian noninstitutionalized population through confidential interviews conducted in households. The NHIS is the nation's largest household health survey, providing data for analysis of broad health trends, as well as the ability to characterize persons with various health problems, determine barriers to care, and compare racial and ethnic populations' health status, health-related behaviors, and risk factors.

Health topics addressed annually include
- Health status and disability.
- Insurance coverage.
- Access to care.
- Use of health services.
- Immunizations (child).
- Health behaviors.
- Injury.
- Ability to perform daily activities.

Additional topics addressed in 2002 include
- Alternative medicine.
- Arthritis.
- Disability and secondary conditions.
- Environmental health.
- Vision and hearing.

National Institutes of Health
www.nih.gov

National Heart, Lung, and Blood Institute

Cardiovascular Disease Research and Outreach Efforts

The National Heart, Lung, and Blood Institute (NHLBI) provides leadership for a national program in diseases of the heart, blood vessels, lung, and blood; blood resources; and sleep disorders. Since October 1997, the NHLBI has also had administrative responsibility for the NIH Woman's Health Initiative.

The Institute plans, conducts, fosters, and supports an integrated and coordinated program of basic research, clinical investigations and trials, observational studies, and demonstration and education projects. Research is related to the causes, prevention, diagnosis, and treatment of heart, blood vessel, lung, and blood diseases and of sleep disorders. The NHLBI plans and directs research in development and evaluation of interventions and devices related to prevention, treatment, and rehabilitation of patients suffering from such diseases and disorders. It also supports research on clinical use of blood and all aspects of the management of blood resources. Research is conducted in the Institute's own laboratories and by scientific institutions and individuals supported by research grants and contracts.

For health professionals and the public, the NHLBI conducts educational activities, including development and dissemination of materials in the aforementioned areas, with an emphasis on prevention.

The NHLBI supports research training and career development of new and established researchers in fundamental sciences and clinical disciplines to enable them to conduct basic and clinical research related to heart, blood vessel, lung, and blood diseases; sleep disorders; and blood resources through individual and institutional research training awards and career development awards. The Institute coordinates relevant activities in these areas, including the related causes of stroke, with other research institutes and federal health programs. Relationships are maintained with appropriate institutions and professional associations; international, national, state, and local officials; and voluntary agencies and organizations.

Each year, the NHLBI assesses progress in the scientific areas for which it is responsible and updates its goals and objectives. As new opportunities are identified, the Institute expands and revises its areas of interest. Throughout the process, the approach used by the Institute is an orderly sequence of research activities that includes

- Acquisition of knowledge.
- Evaluation of knowledge.
- Application of knowledge.
- Dissemination of knowledge.

Several components of the Institute are engaged in research and education activities aimed at the prevention and control of cardiovascular disease (CVD). Highlights of activities are summarized in the following sections.

Division of Heart and Vascular Diseases

The Division of Heart and Vascular Diseases (DHVD) plans and directs a coordinated research program on the causes of heart and vascular diseases and on their prevention, diagnosis, and treatment. Fundamental biomedical research is emphasized. Multidisciplinary programs are supported to advance basic knowledge of disease and to generate the most effective methods of clinical management and prevention. Clinical trials are an important part of the research program; they provide an opportunity to test and apply promising preventive or therapeutic measures.

Research in atherosclerosis encompasses the etiology, pathogenesis, diagnosis, prevention, and treatment of the disorder. Programs include pathobiology and genetics of the vasculature; vascular growth and angiogenesis; interactions of the vascular wall with systemic and humoral factors promoting atherogenesis; and lesion progression, complication, and regression. Targeted areas involve characterization of atherosclerotic plaque prone to rupture, pathogenesis of abdominal aortic aneurysms, the role of homocysteinemia in atherosclerosis, mechanisms of atherosclerosis in various vascular beds, and research on atherosclerotic lesions using human autopsy tissue. Additional studies focus on pathobiological determinants of atherosclerosis, cardiovascular complications of diabetes mellitus, vessel-wall calcification, the role of infectious agents in atherosclerosis, immunobiology of the vessel wall, hormone replacement therapy on atherosclerosis, and effect of protease inhibitors on atherosclerosis development in human immunodeficiency virus (HIV) infection. Of special interest is understanding atherosclerosis risk among minorities.

Studies related to hypertension focus on identifying and characterizing genes involved with hypertension; elucidating regulation mechanisms associated with blood pressure control; identifying causative factors of essential hypertension as well as rare forms of high blood pressure; examining mechanisms by which high blood pressure increases the risk of, or occurs concomitantly with other diseases, such as kidney failure, stroke, diabetes, atherosclerosis, preeclampsia, and left ventricular hypertrophy; and developing preventive strategies as well as novel interventions for hypertension. Additional areas of interest include understanding the biological underpinnings of salt sensitivity; identifying neurological mechanisms responsible for long-term control of blood pressure and functional neurological changes that result in essential hypertension; and understanding the basis of target-organ damage in hypertension. Of special interest is eliminating health disparities among minorities and between men and women.

Basic and clinical studies on arteriogenesis (formation of new arteries), angiogenesis (formation of new blood vessels), and the biology and pathophysiology of blood vessel structure and function in the cerebral, coronary, and peripheral vascular beds are designed to increase understanding of how oxygen, nutrient, and fluid exchange occurs within vessels; how vascular inflammatory response originates and contributes to CVD; how blood flow within the tissues is autoregulated; how vascular smooth muscle contraction is altered; how new vessels are formed; and how vascular remodeling is orchestrated. Scientists are investigating ways to control the inflammatory response in blood vessels, manipulate mechanisms that regulate blood flow, and stimulate the formation of new blood vessels (especially after an ischemic event in the brain, heart, or a limb).

Gene transfer is being used to deliver growth factors to the myocardium to promote development of new blood vessels. Clinical trials are under way to test the safety and efficacy of this approach in humans. Ultimately, these studies should offer insight into developing new therapeutic agents for ischemic disease.

Research in cardiovascular medicine is focused on new strategies to ameliorate disease through improving risk stratification and management and developing novel drugs and therapies. In addition to risk factor reduction, healthy lifestyles and behaviors are emphasized. The preventive and therapeutic potential of nutrition and exercise are currently being evaluated. To date, hormone replacement trials consistently demonstrate lack of benefit with regard to cardiovascular outcomes despite benefits suggested by fundamental and observational data. Devices are used to prevent fatal consequences of ventricular fibrillation in patients at high risk of sudden death, improve ventricular function in heart failure patients with intraventricular conduction delays, and improve survival in selected end-stage heart failure patients who are ineligible for heart transplantation. The development of drug-eluting stents holds promise of significant reduction of restenosis even in patients with a tendency for a hypercellular response to coronary interventions. Current projects encompass developing new strategies for acute and chronic heart disease, cardiomyopathies of different etiologies (i.e., ischemic, valvular, genetic, metabolic, and HIV-related), peripheral vascular disease, aortic aneurysms, and restenosis after percutaneous coronary interventions. Examples of therapies and approaches include diet, exercise, and pharmacologic management of dyslipidemias, genetic susceptibility and directed treatment, diagnosis and management of arrhythmias; surgical and medical management of heart failure; and novel imaging of atherosclerosis. Studies also seek to understand and reduce disparities associated with minority and women's cardiovascular health.

Division of Epidemiology and Clinical Applications

The Division of Epidemiology and Clinical Applications (DECA) plans, directs, and evaluates research on the causes, prevention, diagnosis, and treatment of CVD, as well as on the need for technological development in the acquisition and application of research findings. It supports epidemiologic studies, clinical trials, demonstration and education research, disease prevention and health promotion research, and basic and applied research in behavioral medicine.

Research in the prevention of CVD encompasses clinical trials, community intervention studies, prevention trials, nutrition studies, health education research, and behavioral medicine studies. DECA supports a number of multicenter prevention and education trials to test the efficacy and effectiveness of, and demonstrate the capability of, prevention strategies designed to reduce cardiovascular risk factors. Major studies include determining the effectiveness of school- and home-based interventions to reduce development of CVD risk factors in children, especially those from minority populations; examining the effects of dietary patterns, sodium intake, and other lifestyle factors on blood pressure; and comparing the efficacy of various treatments to prevent major cardiovascular events in adults with diabetes. Studies on increasing the implementation of interventions known to be effective are of particular interest.

Clinical trials are used to evaluate the effectiveness of various medical procedures and therapeutic agents in patients with coronary heart disease, hypertension, and heart failure. Examples include assessing the long-term safety and efficacy of an angiotensin converting enzyme inhibitor to prevent major CVD events in patients with documented normal ventricular function, testing the ability of selected antihypertensive and lipid-lowering drugs to prevent heart attack among individuals at high risk for hypertension and coronary heart disease (CHD), and comparing the use of an implantable cardiac defibrillator to conventional pharmacologic therapy to improve survival among heart failure patients.

Research in behavioral medicine focuses on biopsychologic and sociocultural factors involved in heart, lung, and blood diseases. Areas of interest include central nervous system regulation of the cardiovascular system; identification of psychosocial factors (social support, depression, and hostility) affecting disease etiology, treatment, and rehabilitation; and effects of psychosocial and behavioral interventions on risk factors (smoking, adverse diet, physical inactivity), disease outcomes, and quality of life. Study participants are from all levels of health and from all ages and racial groups.

Investigators are conducting long-term epidemiological studies of heart and vascular, lung, and blood diseases in defined populations in the United States and other countries. These studies focus on the development and progression of CVD risk factors in children and young adults, the development and progression of atherosclerosis measured noninvasively or at autopsy in middle-aged or older adults, and the development and progression of overt cardiovascular and pulmonary disease in older adults. Areas of emphasis include genetic and environmental influences on CVD and its risk factors; trends in incidence, prevalence, and mortality from CVD, stroke, peripheral vascular disease, congestive heart failure, and cardiomyopathy; and relationships between insulin, insulin resistance, and overt diabetes and CVD and its risk factors. Another area of interest is the incidence of and mortality from cardiovascular, lung, and blood diseases. Research strategies apply family, longitudinal, demographic, and vital statistics to study their natural history, etiology, and epidemiology.

Genetic epidemiology has become an increasingly important component of the DECA Research Program. Several long-term studies of twins, multiple generations, Native Americans, and blacks focus on related individuals to estimate heritability and identify genes that contribute to the development of CVD risk factors and CVD. Other long-term studies are storing DNA and testing candidate genes from unrelated individuals. In addition to examining associations between CHD risk factors and development of atherosclerosis, heart failure, cardiomyopathy, and stroke in adults and the elderly, investigators will seek to identify and characterize genes related to CHD and atherosclerosis and to determine how they interact with environmental factors in the development of disease. Additional studies are underway to identify genetic factors influencing coronary and aortic calcification and individual variability in the inflammatory response and to investigate gene-environment interaction, collaborative approaches to linkage analysis, and population screening for genetic diseases.

The research program also focuses on understanding the relationships between insulin, insulin resistance, overt diabetes, and CVD and its risk factors. Scientists are attempting to find and characterize genes linked to risk factors that are associated with insulin resistance syndrome and diabetes. Research strategies include family and longitudinal studies in racially diverse populations.

Office of Prevention, Education, and Control

The NHLBI Office of Prevention, Education, and Control (OPEC) coordinates the translation and dissemination of research findings and scientific consensus to health professionals, patients, and the public, so that information can be adapted for and integrated into health care practice and individual health behavior. To accomplish its mission, OPEC established health education programs and initiatives that address high blood pressure, high blood cholesterol, asthma, early warning signs of heart attack, obesity, and sleep disorders. The programs use two strategies: one focuses on individuals at high risk; the other focuses on the general public. The four largest programs have coordinating committees consisting of national medical, public health, and voluntary organizations and of other federal agencies. These committees help to plan, implement, and evaluate program efforts in professional, patient, and public education.

The National High Blood Pressure Education Program (NHBPEP) was initiated in 1972 to reduce death and disability related to high blood pressure through professional, patient, and public education programs. It is a cooperative effort among the NHLBI, professional and voluntary health agencies, and state health departments that has served as a model for national health education programs and continues to be adopted by other national and international groups. Special attention is directed to reducing health disparities among people with hypertension.

Since the program's inception, the number of people with hypertension who are aware of their condition has increased fourfold, and four times as many people are receiving treatment and controlling their disease. Data from the National Health and Nutrition Examination Surveys (NHANES) indicate that over the past four decades, mean systolic blood pressure has declined by 10 mmHg and age-adjusted mortality rates from heart disease and stroke have decreased by 50% and 60%, respectively.

The NHBPEP is focused on translating research results to improve medical care outcomes and the public's health. It is committed to raising public awareness of the importance of adopting a heart-healthy lifestyle. Research has identified steps that individuals can take to control their blood pressure and to lower their risk for heart disease. For example, certain dietary habits can decrease blood pressure and can prevent it from rising. The DASH (Dietary Approaches to Stop Hypertension) diet—rich in fruits and vegetables, low in saturated and total fat and cholesterol, and containing low-fat dairy products—has been shown to be beneficial for individuals who have high blood pressure and for those who wish to prevent high blood pressure. Combined with a reduced salt intake, the diet can further lower blood pressure.

In 2002, community and professional activities focused on updating the *Primary Prevention Report*, encouraging communities to hold local events to mark May as National High Blood Pressure Education Month, and redesigning and expanding the *Your Guide to Lowering High Blood Pressure* Web page. The NHLBI initiated the development of a major repositioning strategy, which will include new partners, to enhance its position as the U.S. leader in high blood pressure prevention and control, raise the importance of high blood pressure on the national public agenda, and reach individual audiences by designing activities directed specifically to them.

The National Cholesterol Education Program (NCEP) was initiated in 1985 to educate health professionals and the public about high blood cholesterol as a risk factor for CHD and about the benefits of lowering cholesterol levels to reduce illness and deaths from CHD. From 1983 through 1995, the percentage of the public who had their cholesterol checked rose from 35% to 75%, showing that 70 to 80 million more Americans were aware of their cholesterol levels in 1995 than in 1983. Moreover, in 1995, physicians reported initiating diet and drug treatment at much lower cholesterol levels than in 1983. Major elements of the NCEP guidelines for detection and treatment have become established practice.

NHANES III (1988–1994) data demonstrate that the NCEP's dual strategy—one emphasizing the need for detection and treatment for individuals whose high blood cholesterol places them at increased risk for CHD and the other encouraging heart-healthy eating patterns to lower average cholesterol levels for the general public—has had a substantial effect on measured blood cholesterol levels of U.S. adults. Since 1978, the intake of saturated fat, total fat, and cholesterol among the general public decreased significantly, resulting in an impressive decline in average blood cholesterol levels. The prevalence of high blood cholesterol in the U.S. population has also fallen significantly. Cholesterol levels in adolescents likewise have declined.

In 2002, the NCEP focused its attention on disseminating the new *Adult Treatment Panel III (ATP III) Guidelines* on managing high cholesterol in adults. It developed a Web-based kit of materials derived from the guidelines to support cholesterol education for Cholesterol Month 2002 and throughout the year. An ATP III Opinion Leader Dissemination kit was distributed to influential members of the medical community to encourage them to use the guidelines and communicate their importance to professional colleagues. The NCEP is producing a new patient booklet on therapeutic lifestyle changes based on the ATP III recommendations. Additional activities include developing an action plan for reducing lifetime risk for CHD and convening an international conference on scientific issues that should be addressed in developing cardiovascular guidelines. The NHLBI, the American College of Cardiology, and the American Heart Association issued a clinical advisory on the use and safety of statins—specifically focusing on myopathy—in response to concerns that arose after cerivastatin was voluntarily withdrawn from the market by its manufacturer. The advisory provides reassurance that the benefits of statins far outweigh the risks if patients are properly selected and attention is paid to possible side effects.

The National Heart Attack Alert Program (NHAAP) was initiated in June 1991 to reduce morbidity and mortality from acute myocardial infarction (AMI), including out-of-hospital cardiac arrest, through education of health professionals (e.g., physicians, nurses, and emergency medical services personnel), patients, and the public about the importance of rapid identification and treatment of individuals with heart attack symptoms. In 1997, the program's scope was broadened to include early identification and treatment of individuals with acute coronary syndromes such as unstable angina. Since its inception, the program has taught health care providers in emergency departments and emergency medical services systems about the importance of reducing the interval between a heart attack and treatment. Available treatments, if administered soon after heart attack symptoms start, can save lives and minimize heart muscle damage in heart attack survivors.

In 2001, the NHAAP, in partnership with the American Heart Association, the American Red Cross, and the National Council on Aging, launched a major campaign to urge physicians and health care providers to educate their patients about heart attack risk, warning signs, and steps to survival. As part of the campaign to increase awareness of the need to act fast when someone may be having a heart attack, the NHLBI established its *Act in Time to Heart Attack Signs* Web page with educational materials for health professionals, patients, and the public.

The NHLBI Obesity Education Initiative (OEI) began in January 1991 to inform the public and health professionals about the health risks associated with overweight and obesity. Obesity is not only an independent risk factor for CVD, but also a contributor to high blood pressure and high blood cholesterol and is related to sleep apnea.

In 2002, 50 at-risk communities belonging to the NHLBI Hearts N' Parks project, made a 3-year commitment to create model community-based programs to increase the number of children, adults, and seniors practicing heart-healthy behaviors. The project's goal is to reduce obesity, improve nutritional status, and increase physical activity. The American Dietetic Association, in partnership with the project, is providing nutrition consultation. A *Hearts N' Parks* Web page has been established with information on the program.

The NHLBI Women's Heart Health Education Initiative was launched in 2001 in response to the Women's Health Research and Prevention Amendments, Public Law 105-304, which requires the Institute director "to expand, intensify, and coordinate research and related activities, including information and educational programs, with respect to heart attack, stroke, and other cardiovascular diseases in women." The Heart Truth—a campaign directed at women 40–60 years old and health professionals—was launched in 2002 to increase awareness about heart disease, improve detection and treatment of risk factors by health professionals, and motivate national and community organizations to become involved in heart health education. Special attention is given to minority women who are at increased risk for developing CVD.

As a key part of its response to the *Healthy People 2010* national health objectives, the NHLBI initiated a new funding mechanism to establish CVD educational outreach programs in high-risk communities. The program—Enhanced Dissemination and Utilization Centers (EDUCs)—is a partnership between the NHLBI and local communities to eliminate cardiovascular health disparities and increase quality and years of health in underserved populations. In 2001, the Institute awarded EDUCs to high-risk health service areas in Arkansas, North Carolina, Texas, Virginia, and West Virginia to conduct educational projects targeting populations at greatest risk for heart disease and stroke. Multiple strategies to prevent and control CVD risk factors and to promote heart-healthy behavior have been designed specifically for different age groups, ranging from childhood to adulthood. Six additional EDUCs were awarded to areas in Maryland, Ohio (2), Colorado, Nebraska, and North Carolina in 2002.

A major goal of the Institute is to eliminate health disparities and to increase the quality and years of healthy life of all Americans. Through partnerships with groups that have special ties and access to targeted populations, the NHLBI is extending its outreach and educational activities to underserved communities. The Institute is collaborating with the Baltimore City Cardiovascular Health Partnership on a project that has a two-pronged strategy consisting of a population-wide public education campaign and a targeted subgroup outreach and educational approach to build and reinforce positive cardiovascular health lifestyle skills and behaviors. The targeted population consists of blacks who reside in Baltimore City public housing developments.

The Institute's Salud para su Corazón (Health for Your Heart) Initiative, a community-based heart health program for Latinos, is expanding across the United States. Trained local lay health workers (promotores), applying values and culture of the communities and mobilizing partners, teach people how to reduce their risk of developing CVD. As advocates for change, they have increased the number of Latinos in their communities who are engaging in heart-healthy behaviors. In 2002, the NHLBI and the Health Resources and Services Administration signed an interagency agreement to expand the program to communities along the Texas–Mexico border and along the southern border areas of California and New Mexico.

The NHLBI-Indian Health Service Partnership to Strengthen the Heartbeat of American Indian and Alaskan Native Communities is a collaborative effort to educate three tribal communities—the Ponca Tribe of Oklahoma, the Bristol Bay Area in Western Alaska, and the Laguna Pueblo in New Mexico—about cardiovascular health and to reduce their risk for CVD. In 2002, tribal heart health teams received training on topics related to cardiovascular health, including physical activity, obesity, smoking prevention, nutrition, high blood cholesterol, and high blood pressure, as well as on theories of team building, evaluation, and community interaction and intervention. Since then, they have initiated community outreach education activities on cardiovascular health and disease. In addition, they have developed connections with local organizations to aid them with their missions.

Asian Americans and Pacific Islanders are a diverse and heterogeneous group with varying levels of CVD risk factors, acculturation, and socioeconomic status and with different cultures, languages, immigration histories, and community norms related to health and well-being. In 2002, the NHLBI, along with the Asian and Pacific Islander American Health Forum, conducted health assessments among Americans of Philippine, Vietnamese, and Cambodian heritage to obtain information on their knowledge of and attitudes toward CVD and its risk factors, disease prevention, and health behaviors. The assessments will guide the Institute in its development of culturally and language-appropriate materials and activities for these groups.

National Institute of Neurological Disorders and Stroke

Stroke Research and Outreach Efforts

The National Institute of Neurological Disorders and Stroke (NINDS) is the nation's leading supporter of biomedical research on disorders of the brain and nervous system. The NINDS also supports basic, clinical, and population-based research to identify and study the causes, biology, prevention, early detection, and treatment of stroke. Through years of dedicated study, researchers supported by the NINDS have amassed a significant knowledge base about stroke.

- **Landmark Clinical Studies**

  For the past 25 years, the NINDS has been encouraging and supporting major multicenter, randomized, controlled clinical trials evaluating medical and surgical interventions to prevent and treat stroke. More than a score of trials, involving more than 20,000 participants, have assessed antiplatelet agents, anticoagulants, thrombolysis, carotid endarterectomy, hormone replacement, and psychosocial interventions. This large investment of public research dollars is justified by the huge public health burden caused by stroke, which costs billions of dollars yearly in the United States, and the likely savings in health care dollars garnered by the results of NINDS-sponsored clinical trials.

NINDS-sponsored clinical trials are flagship studies in many areas of stroke, influencing treatment decisions daily in clinics throughout the world. The North American Symptomatic Carotid Endarterectomy Trial (NASCET) and the Asymptomatic Carotid Atherosclerosis Study (ACAS) provided guidance on when carotid endarterectomy is indicated for patients with cervical carotid stenosis. The Stroke Prevention in Atrial Fibrillation (SPAF) I, II, and III trials showed which antithrombotic therapy should be given to prevent stroke in patients with atrial fibrillation.

The NINDS t-PA Stroke Trial resulted in the first FDA-approved acute treatment to reduce disability from stroke. Until the completion of that trial in 1995, physicians had nothing to offer their patients that could reduce brain injury from stroke.

- **Stroke in Minorities**

  Stroke remains the third leading cause of mortality in the United States and a leading cause of adult disability; however, the burden of stroke is even greater among minority racial and ethnic groups because of its higher incidence and mortality in these populations. Initial evidence suggests that African Americans may experience more severe strokes and greater residual physical deficits.

  The NINDS 5-Year Strategic Plan on Minority Health Disparities called for a planning panel and workshop to generate a set of recommendations to guide NINDS efforts in research, research capacity building, and outreach to reduce and eliminate disparities in stroke. A Stroke Disparities Planning Panel was held in June 2002, and a follow-up workshop was held in November 2002 to identify specific research needs and areas of opportunity.

  The NINDS is proceeding along several fronts to reduce or eliminate racial disparities in stroke, including support of a large number of research projects that focus on minorities. Additionally, as a result of the Stroke Disparities Workshop, several new prevention and intervention programs are underway or planned.

- **Outreach**

  The NINDS has been working with investigators, clinicians, and private groups such as the American Heart Association and the National Stroke Association to determine the steps that should be taken to educate the public and the medical community about the need for rapid diagnosis and treatment of stroke. Especially emphasized are the specific benefits of the acute stroke treatment, t-PA. The NINDS organized a historic meeting, a National Symposium on Rapid Identification and Treatment of Acute Stroke, in December 1996. The symposium drew more than 400 professionals representing wide areas of the health care system to draft guidelines on how to treat stroke on an emergency basis. The participants made recommendations for change in five key areas: pre-hospital systems, emergency departments, acute hospital care, hospital systems, and public education. The proceedings from the meeting were published and distributed nationally in an effort to increase the number of stroke patients who can benefit from treatment and the number of hospitals that can offer rapid treatment to their patients.

Building on the enthusiasm and spirit of cooperation generated by the symposium, the NINDS assumed leadership of the Brain Attack Coalition, an umbrella group of several national organizations that work together to launch major stroke education campaigns. The latest effort is called *Know Stroke. Know the Signs. Act in Time.* The *Know Stroke* campaign is a multifaceted public education program designed to raise awareness of the signs and symptoms of stroke and the need to act quickly to seek medical care. It includes public service advertising, media outreach, and community education. Through a variety of voluntary organizations and federal partners, the NINDS has distributed hundreds of thousands of brochures and posters and more than 1,000 community education kits. These organizations are using *Know Stroke* materials in educational sessions at hospitals, senior centers, and other places that serve those at the highest risk for stroke.

As a follow-up to the 1996 symposium, the NINDS hosted a national Stroke Symposium entitled *Improving the Chain of Recovery for Acute Stroke in Your Community* in December 2002. About 400 participants from many organizations attended this meeting, which was designed to address the problem of the relatively few number of patients nationwide who are receiving acute treatment for their strokes. Both the American Stroke Association and the National Stroke Association were co-sponsors of the meeting. The attendees were to develop workable plans of action to get more stroke patients treated rapidly. The NINDS will publish the symposium task force reports and post them on the Web, in order to provide practical information that can be used by the medical community for years to come. The result will be improved treatment for the nation's stroke patients.

New Programs

- **Specialized Program of Translational Research in Acute Stroke (SPOTRIAS)**

  The NINDS has initiated a new concept called Specialized Programs of Translational Research in Acute Stroke (SPOTRIAS). The objective of this innovative model is to facilitate translation of basic research findings into clinical practice. This is done in settings where patients with acute ischemic and hemorrhagic stroke are evaluated and treated very rapidly after the onset of their symptoms. The intent of the SPOTRIAS is to support a collaboration of clinical researchers from different specialties whose collective efforts will lead to new approaches to early diagnosis and treatment of acute stroke patients. Training and career development will be part of the SPOTRIAS program.

- **Human Genetics Resource Center: DNA and Cell Line Repository**

  To support its mission of reducing the burden of neurological illnesses and to support outstanding investigators funded through its research programs, the NINDS has established a Human Genetics Resource Center: DNA and Cell Line Repository.

  The goal of the repository will be the elucidation of genetic factors associated with neurological diseases, including stroke. Genetic studies of neurological disorders are increasing in number and complexity. Such studies require a large and diverse sample and accompanying information base. Thus, a repository of DNA samples, immortalized cell lines (from which DNA can be extracted continuously), and accompanying clinical and pedigree data is clearly an invaluable resource for the neuroscience community.

- **Stroke Progress Review Group**

  The large body of research knowledge acquired over the years, coupled with new technologies, is providing a wealth of new scientific opportunities. At the same time, increasing research needs and scientific opportunities required that the NINDS determine the best uses for its resources. In order to address these issues and to fulfill a Congressional request, the NINDS set out to develop a national plan for basic and clinical research in stroke. In 2001, the Institute formed the Stroke Progress Review Group (SPRG), consisting of 30 nationally and internationally recognized stroke experts. The SPRG identified topics to be addressed through a large Roundtable Meeting, whose participants identified gaps in stroke knowledge and set research priorities. The SPRG members and other participants of the meeting issued a report reflecting the energy and enthusiasm of the clinical, research, industrial, and advocacy communities for identifying effective prevention strategies and treatments for stroke.

The comprehensive report from this meeting will serve as a guide for planning research in stroke prevention, diagnosis, treatment, and rehabilitation for the coming years.

APPENDIX D: DEVELOPMENT OF A PUBLIC HEALTH ACTION PLAN TO PREVENT HEART DISEASE AND STROKE

In 2001, CDC initiated development of *A Public Health Action Plan to Prevent Heart Disease and Stroke*. The concept of the plan and the process for its development were presented at the First National CDC Prevention Conference on Heart Disease and Stroke on August 24, 2001, in Atlanta. Valuable input was received, especially from the Cardiovascular Health Council of the Chronic Disease Directors (CDD), who identified representatives to join in the planning process. This appendix outlines this process and identifies the many partners who participated.

Organization

The planning process for the *Action Plan* included several key partners, public health experts, and heart disease and stroke prevention specialists in the United States and abroad. These participants were asked to contribute in several ways, including as members of a Working Group, one of five Expert Panels, or a National Forum. The figure illustrates the organizational structure for the planning process, which included CDC Core Staff.

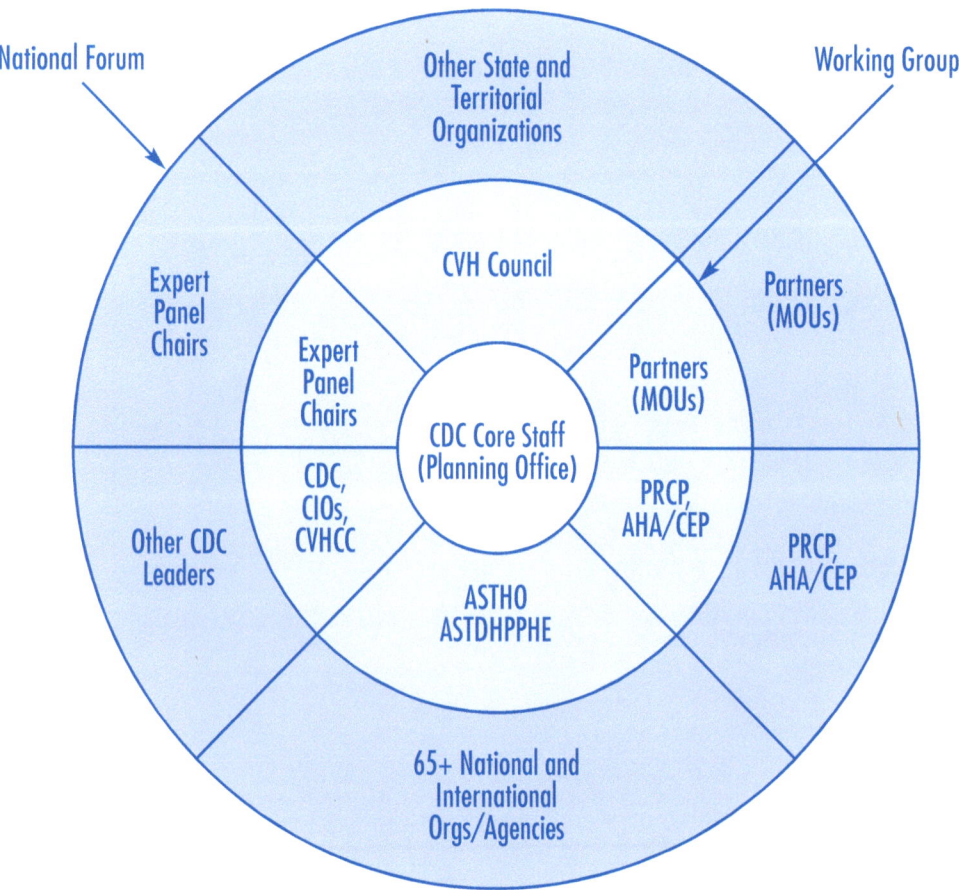

Organizational Structure of the *Action Plan* Planning Process

Note: Abbreviations used in the figure are identified in the text or the participants list.

For the Expert Panels, each of which was chaired by an extramural public health expert, 45 national and international experts contributed to formulation of the recommendations and proposed actions steps. For the Working Group, which also was chaired by an extramural public health expert, 20 national and international experts served. For the National Forum, which was presided over by the chair of the Working Group, 81 individuals representing 66 national and international organizations and agencies other than CDC participated. With technical support from CDC, these groups developed the substance of the plan.

CDC Core Staff

The CDC Core Staff was responsible for coordinating the overall planning process. This staff works for the Associate Director for Cardiovascular Health Policy and Research in the Office of the Director, Division of Adult and Community Health, National Center for Chronic Disease Prevention and Health Promotion, Centers for Disease Control and Prevention (OD/DACH/NCCDPHP/CDC). An outside contractor helped CDC with meeting arrangements and other logistical details.

Expert Panels

CDC convened five Expert Panels, each to address one of the five essential components of the *Action Plan*. The panels identified relevant concerns and problems, proposed solutions, and offered recommendations appropriate to their topics. The Working Group then reviewed these recommendations. The synthesized recommendations are presented in Section 3 of this plan. The corresponding action steps are presented in Section 4.

The titles and topics for the five Expert Panels were as follows:

- **Panel A: Policy and Programs**
  Taking action: Putting present knowledge to work.
- **Panel B: Capacity Development and Support**
  Strengthening capacity: Organization and structure of public health agencies and partnerships.
- **Panel C: Monitoring, Evaluation, and Communication**
  Evaluating impact: Monitoring the burden, measuring progress, and communicating urgency.
- **Panel D: Research in CVH Promotion and CVD Prevention**
  Advancing policy: Defining the issues and finding the needed solutions.
- **Panel E: Global Cardiovascular Health**
  Engaging in regional and global partnerships: Multiplying resources and capitalizing on shared experience.

Each Expert Panel had 16–22 members, including the following:

- Experts from outside CDC nominated from multiple sources and invited to participate on a particular panel based on the specific contribution they would make to the process.
- Members nominated by the Cardiovascular Health Council, CDD, which is part of the Association of State and Territorial Health Officers (ASTHO).
- The Cardiovascular Health Coordinating Committee (CVHCC), made up one or more representatives from each of the five NCCDPHP divisions that deal most directly with cardiovascular health: the Division of Adult and Community Health (DACH), the Division of Adolescent and School Health (DASH), the Division of Diabetes Translation (DDT), the Division of Nutrition and Physical Activity (DNPA), and the Office on Smoking and Health (OSH).

- NCCDPHP's Associate Director for Cardiovascular Health Policy and Research and the CDC Core Staff.

Working Group

The Working Group was responsible for initial critical review of the draft outline of the plan and the development process. Members also formulated the instructions for the Expert Panels, nominated members for the National Forum, and reviewed the final reports of the Expert Panels. In addition, they assessed the proposed implementation process and considered all input from the National Forum in preparing the final document. The 36-member Working Group included the following:

- The chairs of the Working Group and each of the five Expert Panels.
- Representatives from the Cardiovascular Health Council, CDD.
- Representatives from the five NCCDPHP divisions that deal most directly with cardiovascular health.
- Representatives from CDC's National Center for Environmental Health (NCEH) and National Center for Birth Defects and Developmental Disabilities (NCBDDD).
- Each partner working with CDC under a current memorandum of understanding (MOU) in the area of heart disease and stroke. These include one MOU with the American Heart Association (AHA) and American Stroke Association (ASA); the Centers for Medicare & Medicaid Services; the Office of Public Health and Science and the Office of Disease Prevention and Health Promotion, Department of Health and Human Services; and the National Heart, Lung, and Blood Institute and the National Institute of Neurological Disorders and Stroke, National Institutes of Health. CDC also has MOUs with the Ministry of Health and Welfare Canada and with the National Stroke Association.
- Representatives from CDC's Prevention Research Center Program (PRCP).
- Representatives from other national health professional organizations.
- NCCDPHP's Associate Director for Cardiovascular Health Policy and Research and the CDC Core Staff.

National Forum

National Forum participants were responsible for reviewing the draft plan from the perspectives of a wide range of partners, constituencies, and other interested parties. They also were asked to assess priorities for the many proposed action steps and to consider the potential contributions of partners to implementing the plan. The National Forum comprised the following participants:

- All members of the Working Group.
- Representatives from additional state and territorial organizations.
- Additional new partners.
- Additional representatives of the CVH research community.
- Additional CDC staff members from other Centers, Institutes, and Offices (CIOs).
- Other appointees as recommended during the planning process.

General Process and Format

The CDC Core Staff was responsible for overall planning and for executing production of the plan, including preparation of working drafts of all materials and the final draft for publication. The CDC Core Staff established and maintained Internet communications about the process and interim products to make the material widely accessible and to encourage broad-based input. A contractor was responsible for logistical arrangements for all meetings.

The Working Group met first in December 2001 to provide input to the draft outline, draft implementation plan, and Expert Panel instructions and to recommend members for the National Forum. During its second meeting in late May 2002, members reviewed and discussed the reports of the five Expert Panels and the implementation plan. Based on this discussion, the CDC Core Staff prepared a draft of the plan for review by the National Forum.

Each Expert Panel was convened for two meetings, the first during January–February 2002 and the second during March–May 2002. These meetings included preliminary discussions, interim work, and final discussions, which led to completed position papers for each panel that will be published separately.

In preparation for the first meeting, panelists received selected background material and were asked to prepare a written statement on their topics. This material was compiled and distributed to all members of each panel before the meeting. During the first meeting, participants discussed their designated component of the plan and identified approximately five issues of foremost importance regarding that component. This discussion facilitated development of a set of premises, which each panel used as the basis for their recommendations. These premises are as follows:

Panel A: Policy and Programs

- Policy development for cardiovascular health (CVH) promotion and cardiovascular disease (CVD) prevention must proceed under a comprehensive framework that recognizes the full array of cardiovascular disorders (e.g., heart attack, heart failure, stroke, vascular dementia) and the need to establish strategic links with efforts to prevent other chronic conditions of public health concern (e.g., obesity, diabetes, pulmonary disease, cancer).
- For maximum impact, community-wide interventions must address all appropriate settings, all opportunities throughout the life span, and the total U.S. population, with added emphasis on populations at high risk.
- A comprehensive public health strategy must focus on preventing major risk factors and assuring services to detect and control them once they develop. This strategy must also support efforts to widely implement guidelines for early identification and treatment of acute CVD events and prevention of recurrent events.
- The ideal program should be 1) national in scope, with state and local adaptation and implementation; 2) based on strategic partnerships, both innovative and established; 3) comprehensive with respect to CVD development and intervention approaches; and 4) responsive to community concerns.

Panel B: Capacity Development and Support

- Preventing heart disease and stroke requires a robust and effective public health infrastructure. Recent events have underscored the need for improved public health infrastructure in the United States. The current public health infrastructure urgently needs to be transformed to allow initiation of programs that are large enough and have the necessary competencies to achieve the goals of the plan. Such competencies include technical as well as political capacity (i.e., to develop policies, partnerships, and a societal commitment to prevent heart disease and stroke). Both aspects are essential. Technical capacity does not assure its own implementation, and a societal commitment cannot succeed without technical capacity.
- The public health capacities needed to prevent and manage CVD and other chronic diseases differ from those needed for communicable disease control. CVD presents special challenges because of its roots in societal conditions, its protracted duration of

development, its varied manifestations, and the need for a continuum of intervention approaches (from CVH promotion through the full spectrum of primary and secondary CVD prevention). Thus, addressing chronic diseases such as CVD requires an infrastructure of technical expertise and policies different from traditional public health agency models.

- The goals of this plan can best be met by recognizing the needed contributions of a diverse and culturally competent workforce.
- Capacity should be developed specifically to eliminate racial, ethnic, and geographic disparities in heart disease and stroke, through development of resources and competencies that address the causes of these disparities.
- Capacity should be developed at multiple levels, including local (i.e., city, county), state, tribal, and national. Challenges and opportunities unique to each should be considered. All levels should engage communities where people live, work, learn, and play.
- These recommendations can be supported by the accumulated knowledge and experience in public health practice and prevention research, which is sometimes derived from randomized trials but more often depends on other types of evidence (like many public health decisions).

Panel C: Monitoring, Evaluation, and Communication

- Surveillance is needed at national, state, and especially local levels, with indicators established for community and individual measures.
- A strong focus is needed on current and future uses of new data.
- Publicly funded CVH programs must conduct process and outcome evaluations. Privately funded programs should be encouraged to do the same.
- When planning surveillance and evaluation, three questions must be answered: What are the minimum data requirements? What additional data are highly desirable? What is the ideal scope of data collection? These answers are needed to develop appropriate interventions for CVD, to monitor the factors leading to CVD development, and to assess the impact of interventions on the population. These answers are also critical for setting priorities for data collection systems.

Panel D: Research in CVH Promotion and CVD Prevention

- A research agenda for heart disease and stroke prevention must recognize the opportunities for research throughout the life span. Conditions that lead to CVD development (e.g., atherosclerosis, high blood pressure) can result from exposures during childhood, adolescence, or even gestation. Risk factor levels generally progress throughout adulthood. Many older adults remain at high risk for continued progression of atherosclerosis and high blood pressure or recurrence of heart attacks or strokes unless adequate preventive measures are taken. Thus, preventive measures are important in childhood and adolescence (or earlier) and throughout early, middle, and later adult years.
- The concept of best practices is well established in public health and involves systematic review and assessment of available knowledge in accordance with accepted criteria. An appropriate review of the extensive knowledge and experience that already exists from public health practices in preventing heart disease and stroke would advance CVD best practices and help shape the prevention research agenda.
- The distinction between policy, environmental, and individual approaches to addressing CVD should be recognized. All are appropriate, and each has elements especially suited to particular settings.
- New prevention research will continually be needed to identify and evaluate current and proposed interventions, especially those related to policy and environment, which have rarely been investigated. Prevention effectiveness studies are needed to investigate inter-

ventions, addressing such aspects as the percentage of disease occurrence that can be prevented, costs and cost-effectiveness, feasibility (strengths/weaknesses/opportunities/threats), specific target populations, multiple levels (local, state, national), multiple settings (communities, work sites, schools, families), specific behaviors or health states studied as outcomes (e.g., smoking cessation, obesity), and effects of varied combinations of approaches (e.g., in a comprehensive model program).

- Important determinants of cardiovascular risk, including social and environmental conditions, have been investigated much less than personal behaviors (e.g., dietary imbalance, physical inactivity, smoking). These determinants require prominent attention in the research agenda.

- The infrastructure needed for such research includes multiple agencies and organizations at national, state, and local levels (including federal agencies, national voluntary organizations, and foundations). The roles of these and other potential partners in implementing the research agenda are an important aspect of implementing the plan.

Panel E: Global Cardiovascular Health

- A public health strategy for CVH promotion and CVD prevention is guided by commitment to the social values of health as a human right, equity, solidarity, participation, and accountability.[1]

- Cooperating on global CVD control and CVH promotion is imperative and urgent. Partners in this plan recognize the strategic need for strong U.S. involvement in global CVH issues.

- The basic needs of vast numbers of people continue to be unmet, and the resulting health challenges leave many people without hope. A more optimistic view recognizes and responds to the importance of a global context in addressing health and security. Better health—achieved through improvements in basic living conditions, income, education, and social services (including health care)—is a key element to achieving a better and safer world for everyone. Without these elements, better CVH cannot be fully achieved.

- With current knowledge and resources, a world that is substantially free from epidemic heart disease and stroke can be envisioned. Eliminating health inequalities and increasing the quality and years of healthy life are strategic goals for the global community in this century.

- To progress, we must maximize the use of all resources in our globalized, interconnected, and interdependent world. Despite the current picture of world affairs, our commitment to improving health conditions, especially CVH, offers the hope of a better future.

- The first four components of this plan (taking action, strengthening capacity, evaluating impact, and advancing policy) can also apply to global CVH promotion. Global recommendations in these areas must 1) correspond to global needs; 2) correspond to capacities and resources of CDC and its partners; 3) contribute to advancing national CVH or enrich the plan itself; and 4) reflect the underlying values and correspond to the stated vision of the plan.

- Based on the preceding criteria for global recommendations, CDC is assumed to be the primary agency to support their implementation, in conjunction with regional and global partners. The recommendations are directed accordingly.

The second meeting of each panel focused on making specific recommendations for the *Action Plan*. Areas of consensus and difference were identified, and salient points were incorporated in a set of recommendations and corresponding action steps. The recommendations and action steps constituted the primary products of the Expert Panels. These were used to prepare the draft plan, after synthesis by the Working Group.

The National Forum was appointed in spring and summer 2002 and received the draft plan in August 2002. The members met September 4, 2002, to discuss the proposed action steps and the interests of their respective agencies, organizations, and constituencies in implementing the plan. The Working Group then made its final revisions to the draft plan.

Reference

1.	Advisory Board of the First International Conference on Women, Heart Disease and Stroke. *The 2000 Victoria Declaration on Women, Heart Diseases and Stroke*. Victoria, Canada: Advisory Board of the First International Conference on Women, Heart Disease and Stroke; May 8–10, 2000.